Think Eat Cook Sustainably

100 RECIPES,
plus Tips & Ideas for
a Healthy World

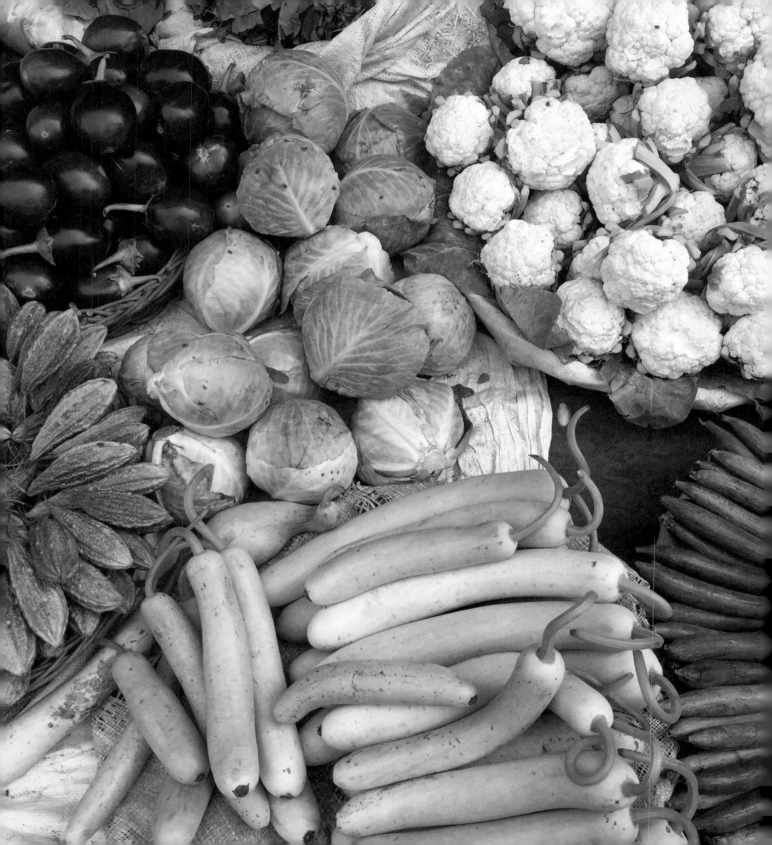

Think Eat Cook Sustainably

100 RECIPES,
plus Tips & Ideas for
a Healthy World

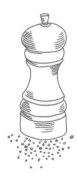

RACHEL KHANNA

Recipe photographs by BLEACHER+EVERARD
Other photographs by Rachel Khanna

Acknowledgements

NO PROJECT IS DONE IN A VACUUM. It is the result of experiences and interactions with many different people and places. The same goes for this book: It is the outcome of concerns, questions, and ideas; of years of learning, reading, and listening; and of visits to farms and farmers' markets, of growing food in the garden, and of tasting different foods and cuisines. At its core, it is the outcome of my passion for healthy food.

I would like to thank my husband and four daughters who encourage me in all my endeavors and who are (almost always) willing tasters for my recipes. As Desmond Tutu said, "You don't choose your family. They are God's gift to you, as you are to them." And so I dedicate this book to my husband Jaideep and our four daughters — Kieran, Anjali, Sophie, and Aaliya — who have been a great gift to me and a continuous source of inspiration. I would also like to thank Susana Mejia who helped me test all the recipes on numerous occasions, and my friend Ali Ghiorse who gave me valuable feedback.

I never tire of working with Teresa Fernandes, whose eye for perfection is unmatched, and who makes it so interesting and fun to create new things. It was also a great pleasure to work with Aliza Fogelson, Enid Johnson, and Nancy Duran, who spent numerous hours editing the book and making sure all my t's were crossed and i's were dotted, and that the thoughts and ideas that swirled in my brain made it onto paper. And it was wonderful to work with Katie Bleacher and Dean Everard, who shot all the beautiful food photography.

– Rachel Khanna

Printed in Turkey
First Printing, 2019
Library of Congress Control Number: 2019947397
ISBN: 978-0-9779568-6-9

Art Director: Teresa Fernandes

Editors: Aliza Fogelson, Nancy Duran

Copy Editor: Enid Johnson

Recipe Photography: Bleacher+Everard

Other Photographs: Rachel Khanna

Illustrations: Janet Stein

Cover Photo: Wild Rice with Black Beans, Peppers & Corn, recipe on page 119

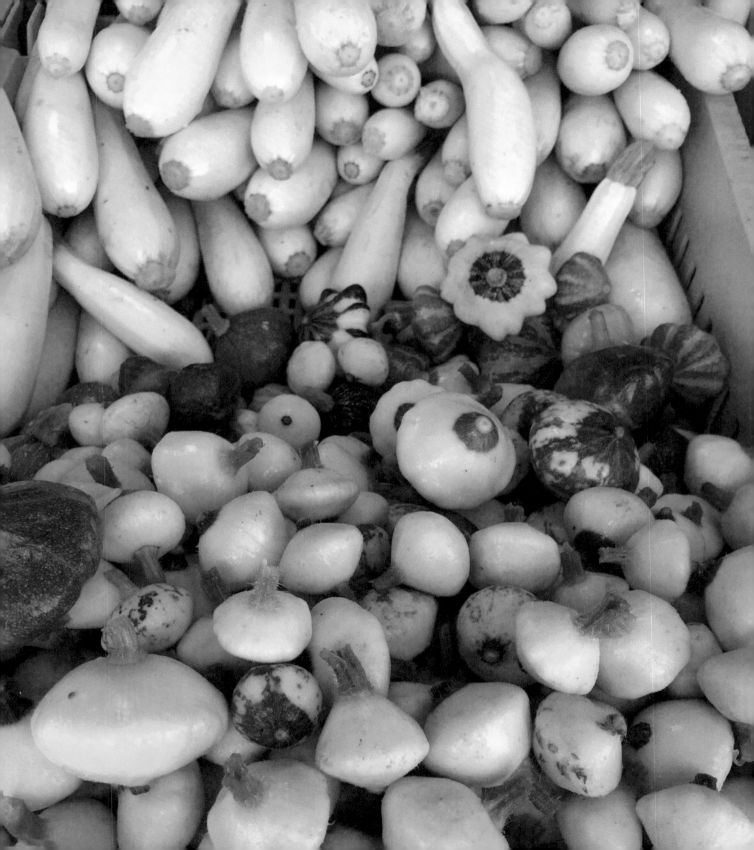

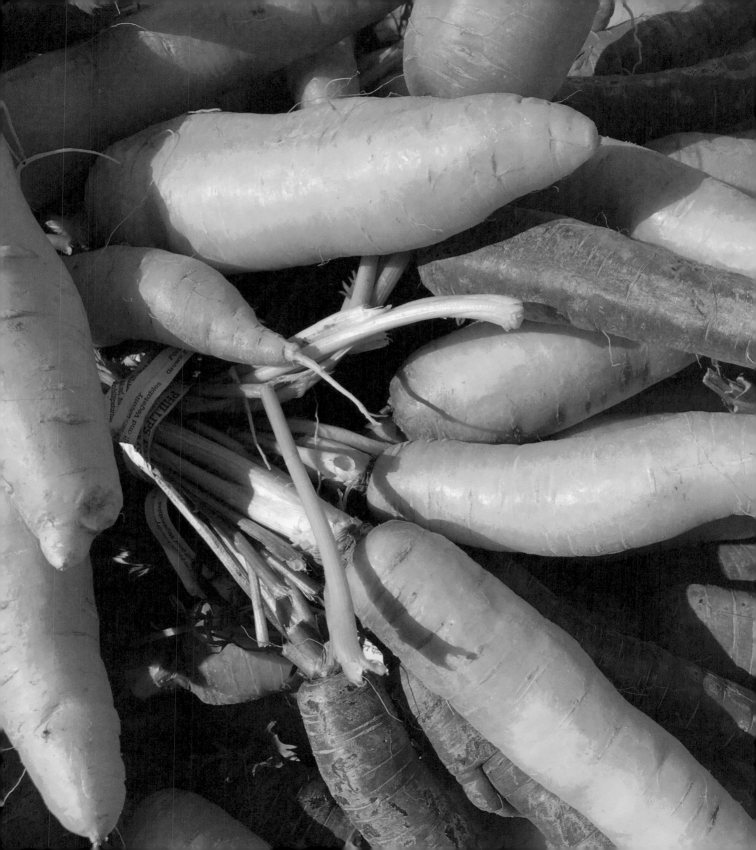

"*If you truly get in touch with a piece of carrot, you get in touch with the soil, the rain, the sunshine. You get in touch with Mother Earth and eating in such a way, you feel in touch with true life, your roots, and that is meditation. If we chew every morsel of our food in that way we become grateful and when you are grateful, you are happy.*"

– THICH NHAT HANH

Introduction

EVERY BITE WE EAT NOT ONLY AFFECTS OUR OWN BODIES AND SOULS, but so too the world at large. This was my conclusion after I completed training to become a chef, where I spent an increasing amount of time learning how to eat for health and balance. Initially, I thought it was sufficient to focus on whole, real foods. But after completing a certificate in integrative health from the Institute of Integrative Nutrition©, and one in food therapy from the Natural Gourmet Institute, I felt like I needed to delve deeper into how the way we eat affects the way we feel. After a few more years of research and reading about food, however, I realized that food is about so much more than that. Yes, food is about health and well-being, but it is also about social justice and the environment. As a result, I wanted to explore a new paradigm to think about the food we eat — one that is more holistic and considers the health of all the organisms that feed the food system. This paradigm is about nourishing yourself while also considering the world — and the other human beings and organisms with which we share it — because, ultimately, we are stewards of this earth.

If we can start becoming more aware about how our food is produced, and where it's coming from, we can create tremendous change for the better, for both our health and that of the environment that nourishes us. I believe it's no longer sufficient to simply say that we are eating lots of vegetables, or that most of the food we purchase is organic. We have to take responsibility for being aware of how an ingredient was produced, by whom (and in what conditions), and what effect its production has on humans, animals, and the environment. We need to consider the workers on the farms, the transport that brought it to our table, and even the smallest microorganisms in the soil.

Why should we care? We are at a critical time — climate change is affecting the world we live in, our soils and water systems have been depleted, and industrial agriculture is threatening our well-being. At the same time, farm

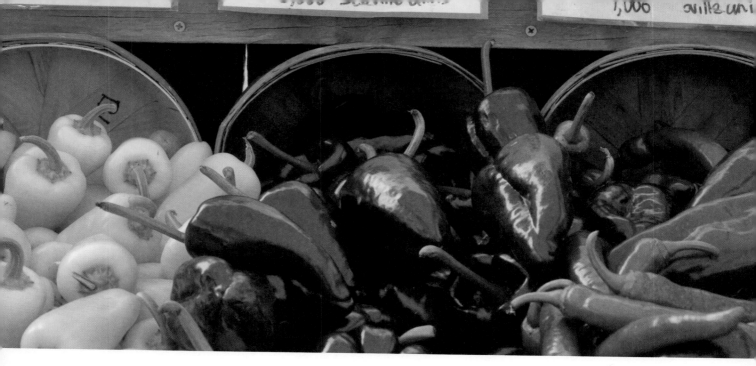

workers are facing lower wages, greater difficulty in finding work, and harder living conditions. But while the idea of eating for both yourself and the world may sound daunting, it's actually a lot simpler than it seems because it really boils down to sourcing food as close to home as possible, thus supporting your local farmers and agricultural workers. In this book, I will explain this in greater detail and offer recipes and tools that represent a more mindful approach to food. The recipes are about eating whole, real foods in season. But they are also about making meals that are simple and delicious, and letting the ingredients speak for themselves.

During the keynote address of a recent food professionals' conference, one of the speakers quoted *Eater's* executive editor, Helen Rosner, as saying that food writing is everything that happens until you swallow, and health writing is everything that happens after you swallow. This book attempts to bridge that gap because everything you swallow will affect how you feel afterwards — physically and emotionally — and will also have a tremendous impact on the world around you.

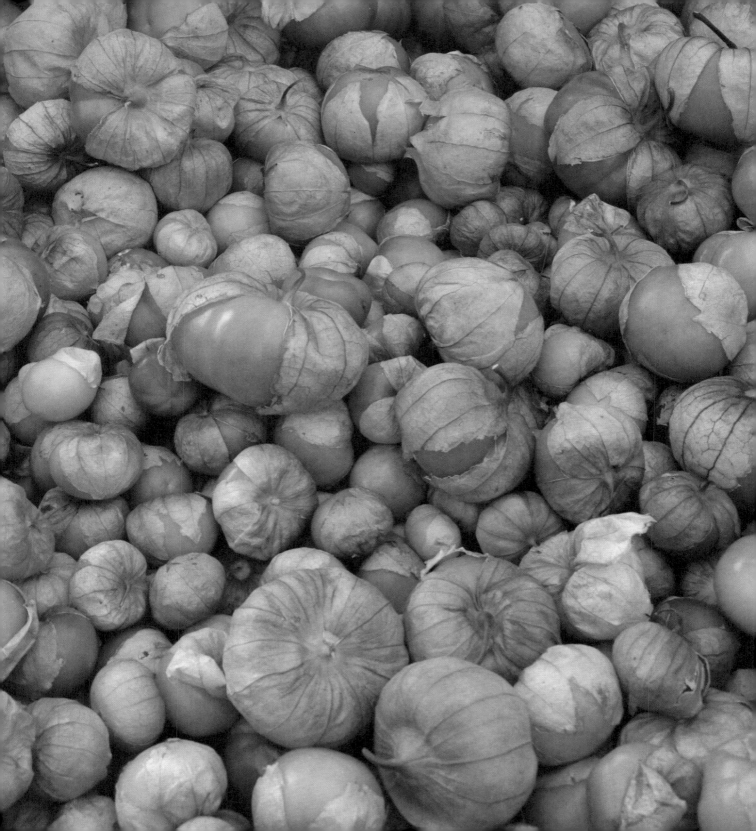

Contents

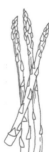
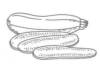

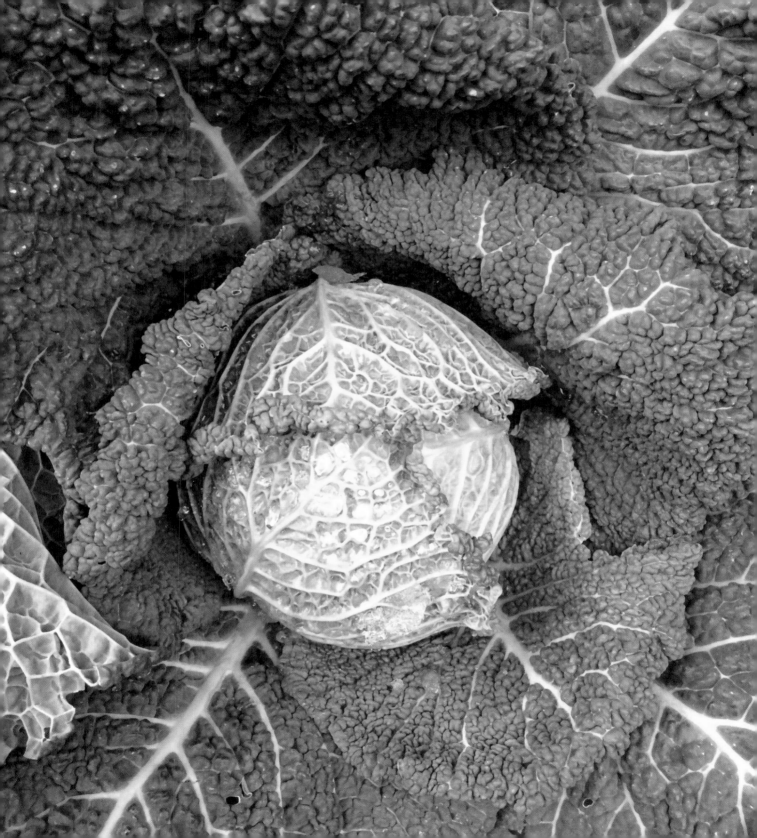

Eating for Yourself & the World

IT IS, OF COURSE, CLICHÉ TO SAY THAT YOU ARE WHAT YOU EAT. Nevertheless, it is true. It is also true to say that you are what you choose to eat. Your food choices should reflect your values as a human being. We should try to eat in a way that nourishes us and keeps us healthy, without depleting the health of others.

Before I ventured into the world of food, I studied political science. As I was discussing my background with some college students recently, it occurred to me that in all these years, I really hadn't strayed that far from my educational background in political science. Eating is a political act. Every choice you make affects the world around you and, in many cases, beyond you. Whether you choose to buy mostly food from local farms or from large industrial farms, these choices have a social, economic, and environmental impact.

According to the World Wildlife Federation, agriculture is the largest cause of habitat and biodiversity loss. Fifty percent of the world's habitable land has been converted to farmland. Agriculture — industrial agriculture in particular — causes the loss of 10 to 12 million hectares (roughly 40,000 miles, or the size of the state of Kentucky) of land to desertification each year; consumes 70% of the planet's accessible fresh water; and is responsible for 14% of greenhouse gas emissions worldwide.[1] Moreover, because we have come to rely so much on a few plant and animal varieties, we are losing genetic diversity in both crops and livestock, which could pose a threat to food security in the future. Bacteria are becoming more resistant to antibiotics, and an infection could easily wipe out a whole species. Another threat to food security is climate change, which is causing plants to have a lower nutrient content. Recent research has shown that as carbon dioxide levels increase, so too does the production of sugars in plants. As a result, the levels of other nutrients diminish.[2] In addition, our food system is one that is built on and fosters economic inequality. As North Carolina chef Andrea Reusing wrote, "Inequality does not affect our food system — our food system is built on inequality and requires it to function. The components of this inequality —racism, lack of access to capital, exploitation, land loss, nutritional and health disparities in communities of color, to name some — are tightly connected. Our nearly 20-year obsession with food and chefs has neither expanded access to high-quality food nor improved nutrition in low-resource neighborhoods."[3] So, clearly, our food choices have an impact far beyond what we may fathom.

The political decision we make when we choose one particular food over another comes down to animal welfare, environmental sustainability, workers' rights, and the support of a local economy. This is our political power as consumers. What follows are a few ways you can make a difference in your own home.

KEY PRINCIPLES

First and foremost, learn where your food comes from and how it was grown.

When we purchase food from large supermarkets and rely on others to make the decisions of where to source foods, we take away our link to farmers and the land. It is so important to create that connection with local farmers so we become aware of where and how the food we eat was grown.

While it's great to get your fruit and vegetables from local (and, if possible, organic) sources, it is paramount to get your meat and poultry from small, humane, and sustainable producers. According to Jonathan Safran Foer in *Eating Animals*, "In a narrow sense it [factory farming] is a system of industrialized and intensive agriculture in which animals – often housed by the tens or even hundreds of thousands – are genetically engineered, restricted in mobility, and fed unnatural diets (which almost always include various drugs, like antimicrobials). Globally, roughly 50 billion land animals are now factory farmed every year. (There is no tally for fish.)"[4] The main reason for factory farming of meat, poultry, and fish is to bring down the cost for consumers. This is done at the expense of animal welfare, the environment, and human health. Safran Foer also notes that, according to United Nations reports, livestock production accounts for 18% of greenhouse gas emissions; excrement from chickens, cattle, and pigs has polluted 35,000 miles of river[4]; and roughly 80% of antibiotics used in the U.S. are for the purpose of meat production. These end up on our plates and in our bodies when we consume factory-farmed meat. This is yet another reason that it's important to eat less meat. One easy solution is to eat smaller portions or have at least two meat-free days a week.

We also need to bear in mind the true cost of food. Local and organic might appear to be more expensive than industrial food but it really isn't. When we purchase industrial food, we fail to account for the taxpayer-funded agricultural subsidies that keep these foods artificially cheap, as well as the long-term cost of depleting the earth's natural resources.

Get produce from sources that help protect the soil rather than deplete it.

We can do better than purchasing organic from large supermarkets. Large-scale producers (both conventional and organic) use farming methods that tend to deplete the soil. Find farmers who are mindful of protecting and enriching the soil. As Dan Barber puts it in *The Third Plate: Field Notes on the Future of Food*, "Wendell Berry once described the land as an 'immeasurable gift,' and he wasn't just referring to food. In the rush to industrialize farming, we've lost the understanding, implicit since the beginning of

1 Source: http://wwf.panda.org/what_we_do/footprint/agriculture/

2 Source: https://www.politico.com/agenda/story/2017/09/13/food-nutrients-carbon-dioxide-000511

3 Source: http://www.npr.org/sections/

4 Source: *Eating Animals*, p.34

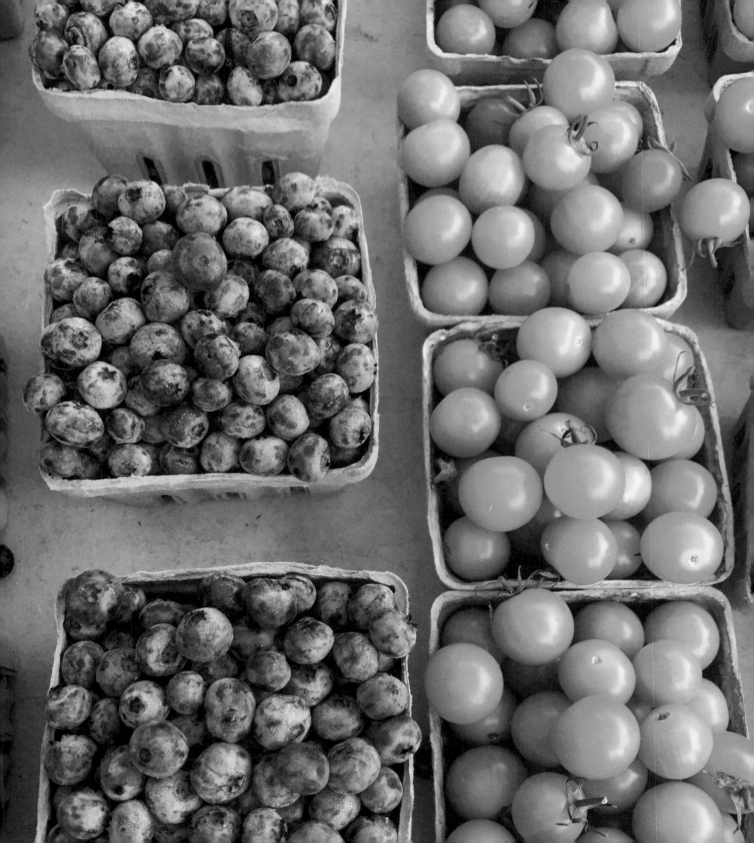

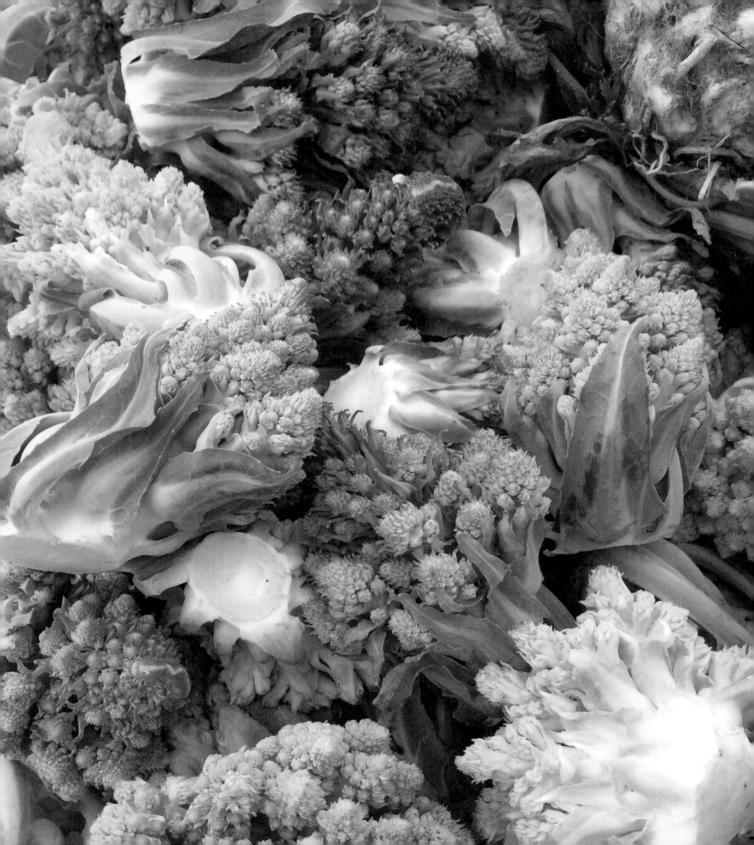

agriculture, that food is a process, a web of relationships, not an individual ingredient or commodity. What Berry refers to as the culture in agriculture is as integral to the process as the soil or the sun."[5] And just as processed foods deplete the bacteria in our gut, industrial agriculture depletes the bacteria needed to maintain a healthy soil, which is critical to all life. The best way to support this culture is by opening the lines of communication with your local farmers and talking to them about what they believe in; visit them at farmers' markets or call them on the phone.

Purchase as many products as possible from local farms or vendors.

I have started to limit my purchases from the grocery store to the bare necessities — mostly grains and legumes. There is a food revolution taking place and it has become so much easier to find food artisans, farmers' markets, CSAs, and farm delivery services that are committed to making and delivering high-quality food. We also need to work to make fresh and healthy foods accessible to more people, and actively support the farms and farmworkers who work to grow our food. In some cases, this may mean visiting local farmers' markets but in others it may mean contacting your elected officials to ensure that legislation supports small farmers and SNAP recipients.

For those of us who live in areas where the availability of produce is limited in winter, opt for domestically grown fruits and vegetables over those coming from across the world. Alternatively, choose canned, fermented, or dried foods from local vendors.

Cut down on waste.

Food waste has a tremendous negative impact on the environment because everything ends up in landfills, and those are large sources of pollution and greenhouse gas emissions. According to a recently published book called *Drawdown: The Most Comprehensive Plan Ever Proposed to Reverse Global Warming,* "...a third of the food raised or prepared does not make it from factory or farm to fork... The food we waste contributes 4.4 gigatons of carbon dioxide equivalent into the atmosphere each year — roughly 8 percent of total anthropogenic greenhouse gas emissions."[6] As consumers, we need to become more aware of how much food we purchase, and try to limit our food waste. Compost as much as possible and eat any leftovers in your fridge.

Become conscious of your own eating.

Just as the health of the environment around us cannot be reduced to a single crop or farming method, so, too, is it impossible to reduce what we eat to one superfood or super-ingredient that has become the latest fad of marketing companies (for more on so-called superfoods, see page 26). Eat a variety of foods and try new things.

In short, this new paradigm means

5 Source: *The Third Plate: Field Notes on the Future of Food,* p. 175.

6 Source: *Drawdown: The Most Comprehensive Plan Ever Proposed to Reverse Global Warming,* edited by Paul Hawken, p. 42.

primarily eating vegetables and whole grains and legumes, and sourcing these as locally as possible. It's about eating from the ground up and being aware of your environment and the environment that your food is grown in. Just as good health relies on having a balanced ecosystem in the body, so, too, does producing healthy food mean supporting and nourishing the soil. We need to become conscious of this process by building relationships with our food providers, learning their principles, and supporting farmers and food producers who are mindful of how the food they produce affects the earth. Ultimately, by doing so, we will reap the benefits of better food. It means spending less time at the supermarket and more at the farmers' market sourcing produce, meat, and poultry that is sustainably raised or farmed.

Contact your legislators and elected officials.

Our elected officials have a duty to represent our interests in government and we have tremendous power as voters. Do not be afraid of letting them know what your thoughts are, especially when it comes to food, farming, and the environment. The National Sustainable Agriculture Coalition (**www.sustainableagriculture.net**) has a great website with specific actions to take to contact legislators about sustainable farming.

THE NEW EATING PARADIGM

It's clear that eating a diet rich in whole, real foods keeps us healthy. Here's what that means, practically speaking. These are some ground rules for you and your family to live by:

Consume lots and lots of fruits and vegetables.

You can never get enough fruits and vegetables. They are loaded with important vitamins and minerals, plus a key element that we tend to forget about—fiber, which helps feed the good bacteria in our gut and keeps us feeling satiated.

There are more than 100 trillion microbes residing in our bodies, and most of them are in the intestines. So, it's not surprising that gut health has surfaced as a topic of discussion. Eighty percent of our immune system resides in our gut too, so, naturally, the health of our gut is paramount to ensuring our well-being. More recently, researchers have found that gut health is a key factor in weight loss, mental and emotional health, and brain development. The balance of good and bad bacteria in our body also helps regulate its inflammatory responses, which may in turn reduce the rampant, chronic inflammation that is a big factor in many modern diseases.

The problem is, we've slowly been eliminating the good bacteria from our bodies in the following ways: we don't eat as many fermented foods with good

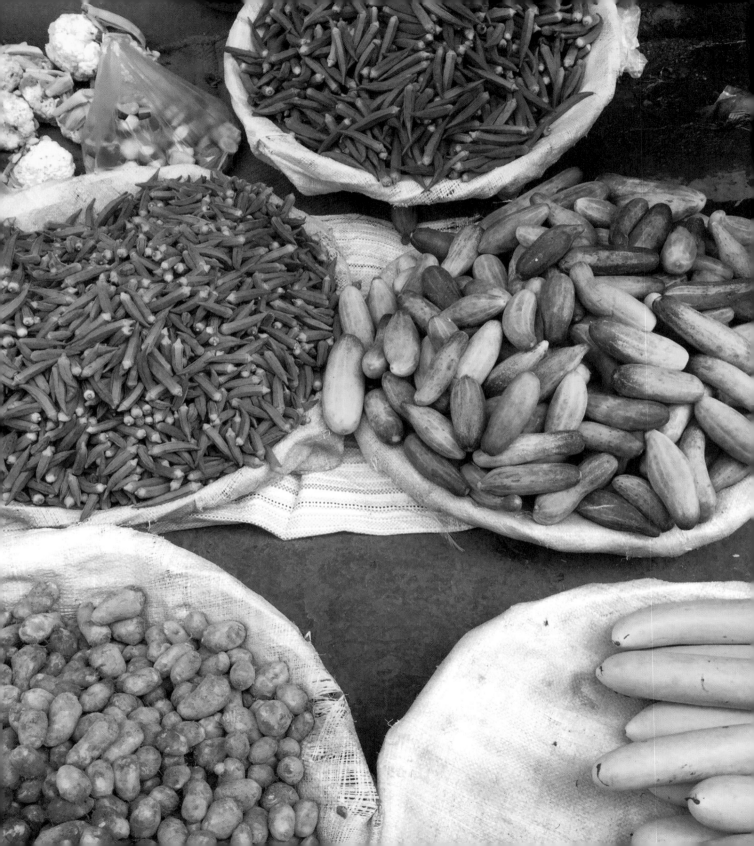

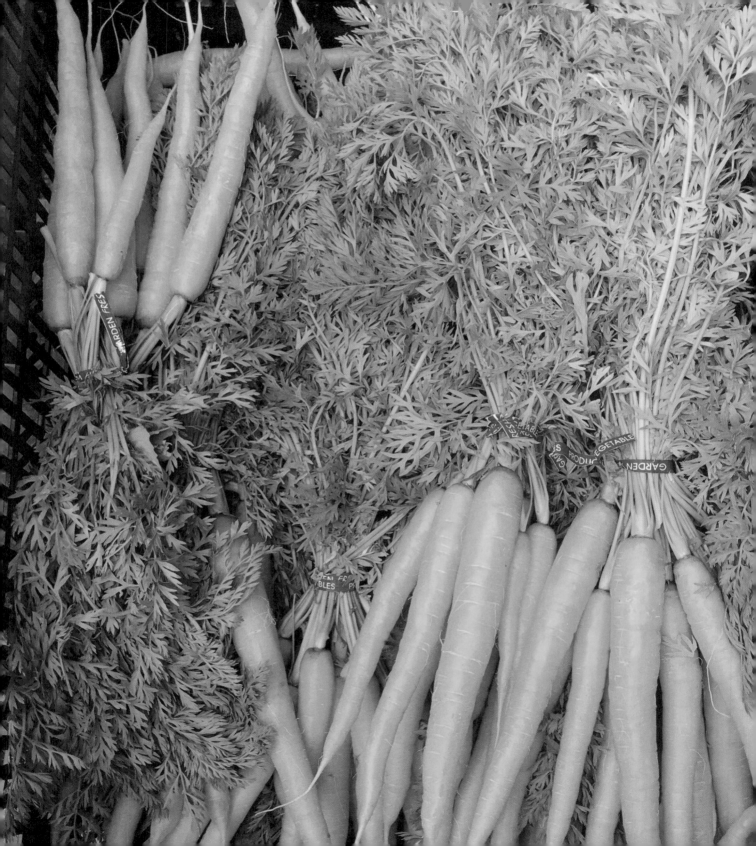

bacteria as we used to (think: sauerkraut, kimchi, yogurt, kefir, pickles, kombucha, miso, and tempeh); we use too many antibacterial cleansers and over-sanitize everything, so our bodies no longer know how to fight off infection; antibiotics are used widely in our food production and this exposure decreases our resistance to bacteria; we have a high-sugar diet, which feeds the bad bacteria; and we are under constant stress, which suppresses our immune system.

Eating lots of fruit and vegetables can help regenerate the good bacteria in our gut, flush out environmental and other toxins that we are exposed to, and strengthen our immune system. In short, they nourish us in better ways than processed foods do.

From an environmental standpoint, eating lots of different fruits and vegetables creates a variety of crops, which, in turn, ensures genetic diversity. A diverse plant and animal gene pool can provide protection from disease and other environmental changes.

Choose healthy sources of protein, such as grass-fed meats and dairy products, pasture-raised poultry and eggs, and organic, sustainably sourced fish.

In this area, it is especially critical to make the right choices, both for yourself and for the environment. Factory-farmed animals live in inhumane conditions and are poorly treated. They rank as one of the top causes of antibiotic resistance worldwide, and, in the case of meat production, are a large

contributor to greenhouse gas emissions. This is why it is crucial to source locally produced, 100% grass-fed, and pasture-raised meat and poultry.

Approximately 80% of antibiotics used in the United States are given to factory-farmed animals that don't necessarily need them. As Maryn McKenna notes in *Big Chicken: The Incredible Story of How Antibiotics Created Modern Agriculture and Changed the Way the World Eats,* as chicken production increased so did the use of antibiotics as growth promoters, and to treat illness. Indeed, expanding chicken production and breeding them to have specific traits that consumers want has led to weak chickens rife with diseases. All these antibiotics end up in the environment when they are excreted by the chickens as waste. McKenna writes, "…manure is the source of much of the resistant bacteria that spread from farming…(But) while animals are being raised, the bacteria in their guts — and any unmetabolized antibiotics that their bodies did not absorb — pass out of them into chicken house litter, or the vast pits or ponds of liquid manure on pig farms and cattle feedlots. When that manure is disseminated through the environment…the bacteria it contains spread too."[7] This explains why we have seen a drastic rise in human resistance to antibiotics — so much so that the World Health Organization considers it one of the biggest threats to global health, food security, and development today.

Furthermore, meat and dairy production releases huge amounts of methane, a greenhouse gas that is one

7 Source: *Big Chicken: The Incredible Story of How Antibiotics Created Modern Agriculture and Changed the Way the World Eats,* Maryn McKenna, p.168.

of the main causes of climate change. This is especially the case for cattle that are fed a diet of corn and soy because they can't digest it and end up producing excessive amounts of gas. Finally, the business of industrial meat production is one of the most unfair and dangerous for workers, many of them migrant workers or refugees. They spend long hours in unsafe conditions where it is not uncommon to encounter accidents or suffer from chronic physical injuries.

When it comes to dairy, many people have developed allergies to dairy products. The reason is that the lactase in milk — an enzyme that makes it digestible — is removed during the homogenization and pasteurization of milk products. Moreover, conventionally processed milk and milk products are produced with the addition of hormones and antibiotics, which eventually make their way into our glasses or onto our plates. This is why I prefer to drink and eat organic and raw milk and milk products whenever possible.

With regards to fish, the problem is two-fold. On the one hand, marine capture production (as opposed to aquaculture — or fish farming — production) has led to severe overfishing of many fish populations. According to the UN Food and Agriculture Organization's 2016 report on the State of the World Fisheries and Aquaculture, "Based on FAO's analysis of assessed stocks, the share of fish stocks within biologically sustainable levels has exhibited a downward trend, declining from 90 percent in 1974 to 68.6 percent in 2013. Thus, 31.4 percent of fish stocks were estimated as fished at a biologically unsustainable level and therefore overfished."[8]

On the other hand, fish farming destroys coastal wetlands communities and can introduce diseases into non-farmed fish populations. In addition, farmed fish are the equivalent of meat and poultry produced on factory farms — they are fed unsuitable diets, loaded with antibiotics, and raised in overcrowded, unsanitary conditions.

If you do choose to eat meat, poultry, dairy, or fish, the key is to source them well and make sure they are sustainably raised. Here are a few things to think about:

- **Consider quality over cost.** Pay a little more, eat a little less, but eat better.

- **Eat more underutilized cuts of meat** or poultry, or underfarmed fish. This helps small farmers and fishermen stay in business and produces less waste.

- **Eat a heritage species.** As Patrick Martins puts it in The Carnivore's Manifesto, "The viability of the livestock population depends on a strong genetic base. Novel pathogens, natural or man-made, can wipe out one variety while having no effect on another; which means that relying on only one or two is dangerous — we have to keep rare and heritage breeds viable by creating an active market for them."[9] This applies to poultry as well.

8 Source: http://www.fao.org/3/a-i5555e.pdf

9 Source: The Carnivore's Manifesto, p.6

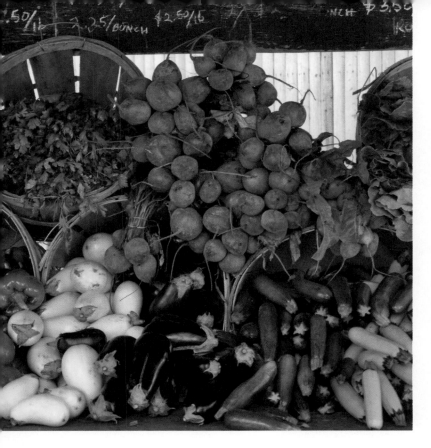

As far as gluten is concerned, there has been a lot of debate on whether people should eat gluten or not, regardless of whether they have celiac disease (a disease in which the intestine is sensitive to gluten and prevents the body from absorbing other nutrients). Unless you are celiac, moderation is best— as with most things in life. I limit my intake of wheat products to once or twice a week, and opt for gluten-free grains, such as rice, quinoa, oats, and corn, for other meals throughout the week. When possible, I try to bake with nut flours, rather than wheat flours.

When I use grains that contain gluten, I try to choose those that are less refined, such as farro or barley. What I do caution against is using gluten-free substitutes, which often contain a lot of sugar and refined starches. I also don't recommend eating much rice because rice farming is actually one of the larger producers of methane, a greenhouse gas responsible for climate change.

Opt for whole grains and legumes (beans).

If we are to eat less meat, we need to ensure that we are getting enough protein. Other than meat, poultry, and fish, the best sources of protein are grains and legumes. When grains and beans are combined, they create a complete protein. Whenever possible, try to eat whole grains because they are not refined and — most important — they contain fiber which, as I noted earlier, is so crucial to gut health. Luckily, there is a wide variety of grains and legumes and it is easy to use them interchangeably. I find grains particularly useful for warming the body in winter, or for vegetarians seeking good sources of protein.

Try to get foods that have an expiration date, that don't come in a box, and that won't stay in your pantry for months at a time.

This means cutting out the processed stuff — there's nothing good in any of those so-called "foods." Processed foods are loaded with sugars and preservatives to help them stay on the shelves for extended amounts of time. As a result, they are devoid of key nutrients and vitamins, especially fiber.

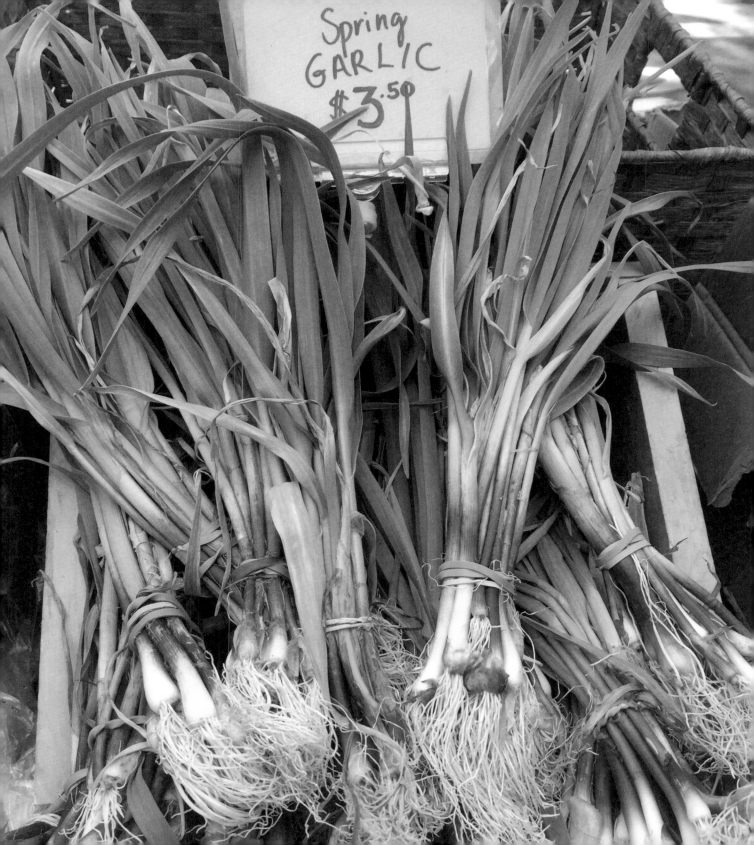

SOME BASICS

1. Choose local before organic, ideally from your farmers' markets or CSAs.

I prefer to choose local ingredients over organic ones, simply because I like to support small, local farms. I feel better supporting these farms rather than large industrial operations (even organic ones), which tend to use intensive farming methods that can deplete the soil. We are quickly losing touch with the way food is grown and need to encourage these local farmers who spend their time growing the best produce for us to eat. Because organic certification can be costly, many farmers are not certified even though they choose no-spray or low-spray farming methods. It's definitely worth a conversation with the farmer.

2. If you have to go to the supermarket, stay on the perimeter.

That's where all the freshest ingredients are — the fruit and vegetables, meat, and fish. Anything in the interior aisles has been processed and may contain artificial ingredients or preservatives. If you do venture into the center aisles, try to purchase products that don't have an extensive ingredient list or an expiration date that is years away. In general, I like to follow the 80/20 rule — 80% fresh and 20% packaged foods.

3. Avoid Genetically Modified Organisms (GMOs).

Organic fruits and vegetables have a product code that begins with 9; conventional produce has a product code that begins with 3 or 4; and genetically modified foods (GMO) have a product code that begins with 8. However, even this system can be misleading because the GMO label is optional. Produce that is typically genetically modified includes papaya from Hawaii, some zucchini and yellow squash, and some corn on the cob. Many processed or packaged foods contain ingredients that have been genetically modified as well. In particular, foods containing soy, corn, wheat, canola/rapeseed, sugar and sugar beets, and dairy are most likely genetically modified unless stated otherwise. The main problem with GMOs is that they may cause genetic changes that are unexpected and potentially harmful to us.

4. Minimize purchases of packaged and frozen foods.

A packaged or frozen food that is organic isn't necessarily healthy. Often, packaged or frozen foods — organic or otherwise — have a lot of additives, preservatives, and sugar to enhance the flavor and keep the food on the shelf for extended periods of time. Again, if a product has a long list of unpronounceable ingredients, chances are it's not good for you.

5. Experiment with new ingredients.

It's so easy to fall into a rut and prepare the same meals over and over again. I know — I do it all the time. Once in a while, purchase a new ingredient and try a new recipe, or cook your way through this book. This will make shopping and cooking fun!

Here are a few reasons it's good to give new ingredients a go:

- They say that variety is the spice of life — experimenting is a great way to keep things interesting in your kitchen and at the dinner table.

- New ingredients expose you to a range of nutrients and vitamins that may not be in the foods you typically eat.

- You'll set an example for your kids, which may encourage them to try new foods, too.

TREND OR TRIED-AND-TRUE?

We often hear about quick-fix ways to improve our health: superfoods, juicing, or various forms of elimination diets. It seems like every few months there is a new buzzword. All the hype is designed to give you the impression that there is a magic food that will make you live longer, feel better, and look better. In general, I find that none of these substitute for a well-rounded diet of whole foods.

SUPERFOODS
I regularly see articles stating the benefits of particular phytonutrients, vitamins, and minerals in food.

Broccoli and cabbage can help boost a person's memory, blueberries can help lower blood sugar, sea vegetables can help the liver…. But research has shown that we can't look at foods for their individual health properties. In general, we need to have a more holistic perspective on food. I don't believe there is such a thing as a "superfood," and I find the whole concept to be misleading.

According to a CNN report, the term "superfood" was coined by Dr. Steven Pratt in 2004. As the article states, "According to Pratt, a superfood has three qualifications: It has to be readily available to the public, it has to contain nutrients that are known to enhance longevity, and its health benefits have to be backed by peer-reviewed, scientific studies."[10] The idea is misleading because it gets people thinking in terms of specific elements that are or are not beneficial to us. Instead, we should be focusing on an overarching philosophy of eating real food, not just about eating fats, vitamin C, or magnesium. We need to eat a variety of nutrients — carbohydrates, proteins, and fats — as well as a whole host of different vitamins and minerals (some more than others at various times). These are found in different combinations in all vegetables, fruit, whole grains and legumes, nuts, dairy products, poultry, fish, and meat, which is why a balanced diet is key. Moreover, we have to be wary of the information we receive because research extolling the benefits of one food is often funded by the

10 Source: http://www.cnn.com/2012/04/10/health/super-foods-weight-loss-diet/

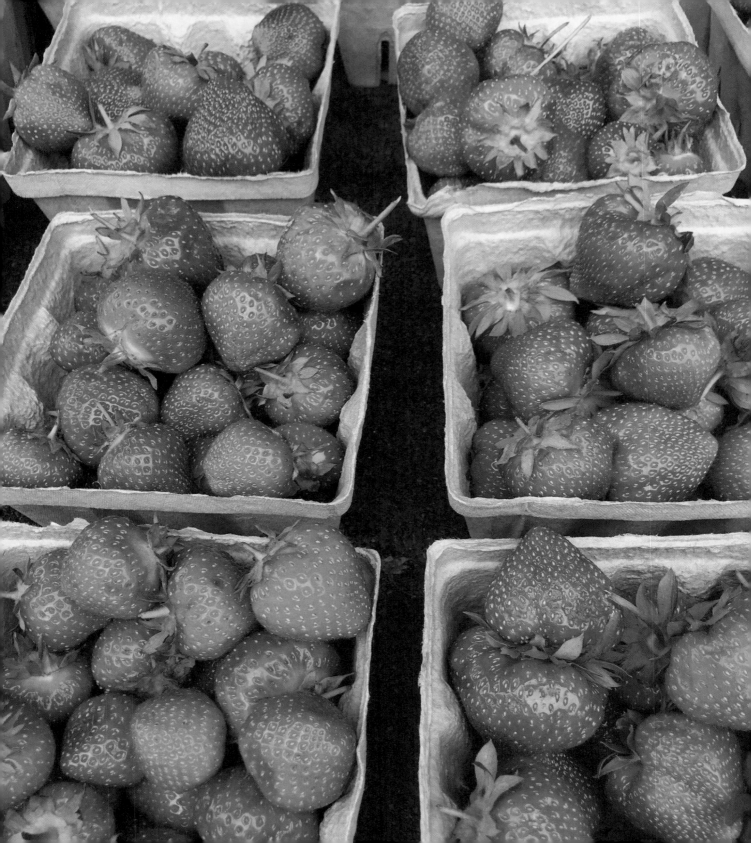

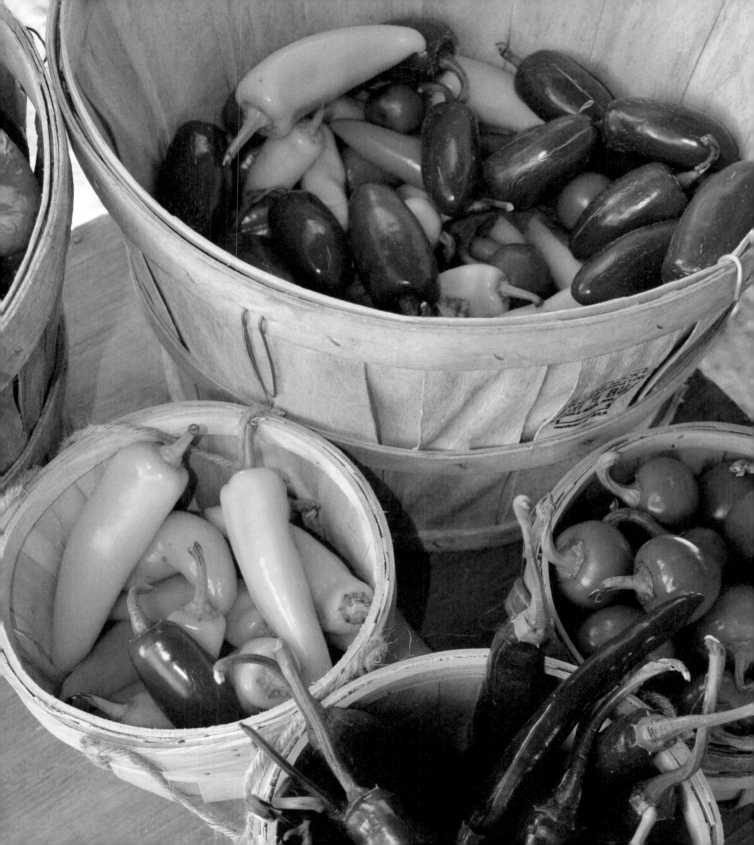

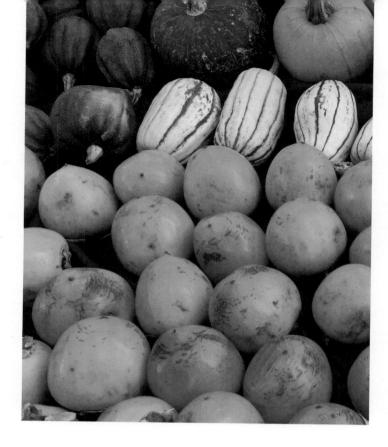

needs. Our lifestyles vary, as do our environmental conditions. And we don't all evolve in the same way. Instead of approaching our diet with the question, "How will what I eat today fill my body's requirements for x or y nutrients or vitamins?," a more helpful question is, "What are the (real) foods that will provide the best nourishment for my body at this moment in my life?"

MEAT ALTERNATIVES

One of the key ways to mitigate climate change is to reduce (or stop) one's consumption of meat. Recently there's been a lot of buzz around meat alternative products. And, while I've given these a lot of thought, I have to say that I am not a fan for several reasons. First of all, if our goal is to encourage people to eat less meat then we should be focusing on a plant-rich diet, not trying to create alternatives to meat. Secondly, Some meat alternative products are made with genetically modified soy. Soy farming is a large cause of deforestation, which is a large emitter of carbon, and genetically modified soy is grown with a chemical that contains glyphosate, a known carcinogen. Finally, most meat alternative products are made by isolating proteins and nutrients from plants and legumes. In other words, they are made with parts of whole foods but not whole foods and, at the end of the day, they are really processed foods.

industry producing that food. As Marion Nestle notes in her book, *Unsavory Truth: How Food Companies Skew The Science of What We Eat*, "Foods are not drugs. To ask whether one single food has special health benefits defies common sense. We do not eat just one food. We eat many different foods in combinations that differ from day to day; varying our food intake takes care of our nutrient needs. But when marketing imperatives are at work, sellers want research to claim that their products are "superfoods," a nutritionally meaningless term. "Superfoods" is an advertising concept." ‖

Finally, each one of us is different. We all have distinct constitutions and

‖ Source: *Unsavory Truth: How Food Companies Skew The Science of What We Eat*, p.76.

JUICING

There's a misconception that all foodies and health nuts are crazy about juices. I for one am not an enthusiast. Juices contain too much sugar and not enough fiber, and they aren't very satisfying. In terms of our health, juices are a very concentrated form of sugar. The problem is not the sugar per se but the fact that without the fiber to accompany it, the sugar is rapidly absorbed into the bloodstream, producing a sugar rush. When we consume too much sugar, the excess energy produced gets stored as fat and eventually causes weight gain. The lack of fiber in a juice also limits the good bacteria in our gut. Bacteria thrive on fiber, and this is why it is so much better to eat the whole fruit rather than just the juice.

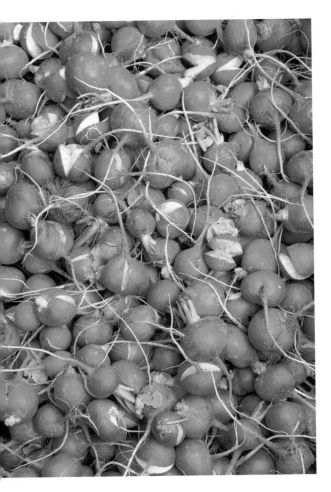

In terms of the environment, juices (cold-pressed juices, specifically) aren't great either. According to a recent article in *Modern Farmer* magazine, a 16-ounce juice produces 3.5 pounds of pulp waste, which can't even be used in compost. In 2015, 175,000 tons of pulp waste ended up in landfills. Once there, the pulp rots and produces methane gas. So, for 175,000 tons of pulp waste, the equivalent of 200,000 tons of carbon dioxide is emitted into the atmosphere — a big problem for the environment.[12] Smoothies are slightly better because nothing gets wasted, though they also tend to have a lot of sugar.

I much prefer soups to juices because they do contain fiber, in addition to all the nutrients and vitamins that juices provide. They are also easy to digest — so the body can easily absorb all the healthful properties— making them especially useful when someone's immune system is compromised. And, best of all, they create very little waste because the entire vegetable can be used. Soups are also a good way to use overripe or less attractive vegetables.

12 Source: https://modernfarmer.com/2016/06/cold-pressed-juice-food-waste/

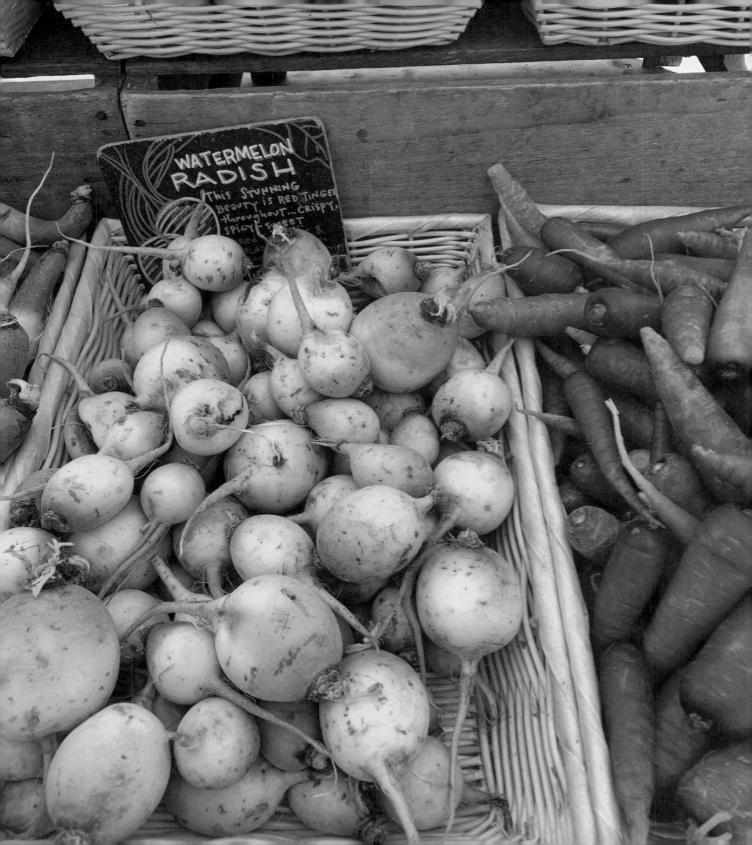

WATERMELON
RADISH
this STUNNING
BEAUTY is RED TINGE
throughout...CRISPY
SPICY+ SWEET...

ELIMINATION DIETS

What are known as elimination diets used to be recommended by physicians to help assess whether patients were suffering from food allergies. And recently they've become a trend. They require you to remove the carbs, grains, legumes, or dairy, or take out foods that contain certain proteins.

I find that these are highly restrictive when the focus in eating should be on making holistic choices that affect our lifestyle and the world around us. Eliminating certain types of food (carbohydrates, meats, fats, etc.) will never be as effective as finding the right combination of real foods that suit us in a particular moment. We need a mixture of protein, carbohydrates, and fats to help us survive. Our bodies don't recognize refined or processed foods, artificial sweeteners, or dietary supplements as foods meant to nourish us. And they don't.

Whole, real foods nourish us on multiple levels — both physical and emotional — while fake foods (such as processed or refined foods, or foods with added sugars) deplete us. They take away nutrients from our body, in turn weakening our immune system. The recipes in this book are designed to provide the nourishment and energy our bodies need. And because time is of the essence for most of us, I've tried to keep the recipes simple, and — where possible — I've provided general guidelines for easy variations.

I am not a fan of diets and this is not a diet book. Instead, this book offers a mindset on how to approach food. I've included 100 recipes that focus on whole, real foods instead of processed ones, featuring easy-to-find ingredient lists. The focus is on maximizing the intake of fruits and vegetables, incorporating whole grains, and limiting (but not necessarily eliminating) meat, poultry, and fish products.

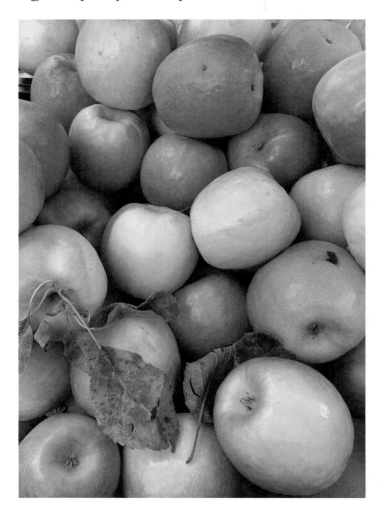

GETTING YOUR FAMILY INVOLVED

Following these few simple steps can create a lifetime of healthy habits.

1. Eat dinner together.

If the kids are home, then we are eating together. This is something that has always been really important to me, especially as my children have gotten older, because it ensures that all of us reconnect as a family. Plus, it provides an opportunity to model healthy behavior and encourages a long-held healthy-eating lifestyle.

2. Go to the farmers' markets.

My husband and I love going to the farmers' markets with our children because they have the opportunity to see what is growing at that time of year or in that part of the world. They also get to interact with farmers and choose foods that appeal to them.

3. Include your family in the meal planning and cooking.

While family meal planning may sometimes start a lively debate on the weekly menu, it is a good way to make your family feel some "ownership." Better yet, get your family involved in the cooking. When we are on vacation, I delegate specific tasks to each child (chopping some herbs, making salad and dressing, or grating cheese). This way, I have help getting dinner on the table quickly and everyone feels like they had a hand in the meal. And, they are learning a vital life skill—cooking!

4. When you travel, take cooking classes together.

It is such great fun to take cooking classes as a family! If it is possible to do so when traveling, I highly recommend signing up for cooking classes at local facilities.

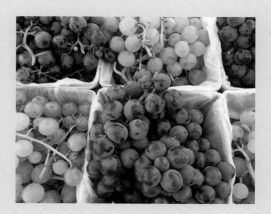

What follows are creative and healthy twists on classic recipes, providing you with some new fundamentals. Highlighting seasonal and nutritious ingredients, tried-and-true techniques, and innovative flavor combinations, these recipes will become mainstays in your household. In each section, I've also provided a "formula" for a signature dish, demonstrating the methods and variations you'll need to master the recipe. »

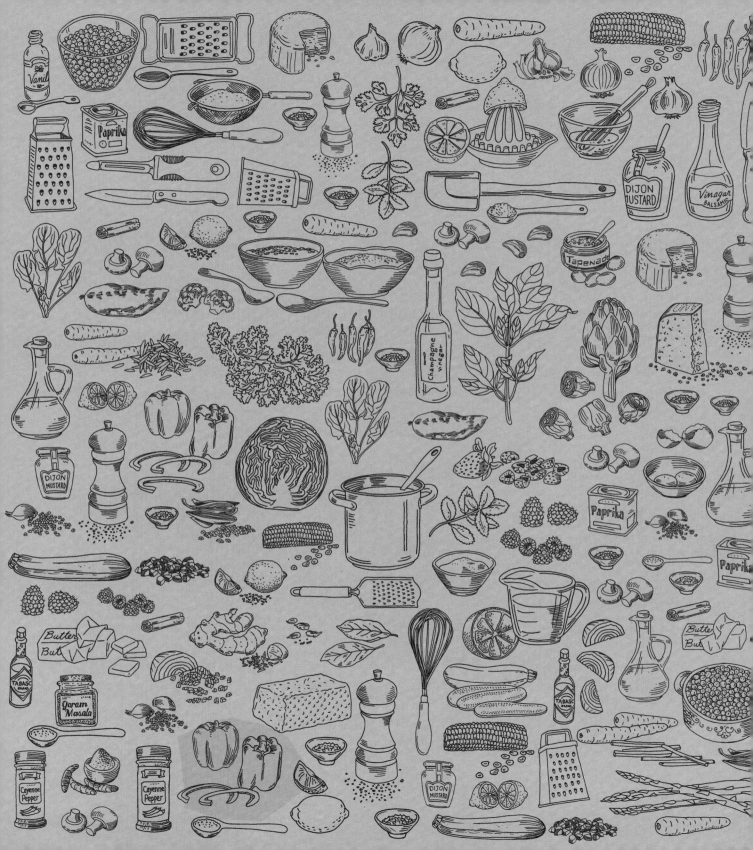

RECIPES

Breakfast & Brunch

What's nice about breakfast and brunch is that there is such a wide variety of food options, ranging from savory to sweet. In our house, breakfast is always a little tricky because everyone has different preferences and time is of the essence. So, short of making six separate meals for the six of us, I try to find recipes that appeal to everyone. Here are some of my healthy favorites.

Beginner's Bread, recipe on page 39 ▸▸

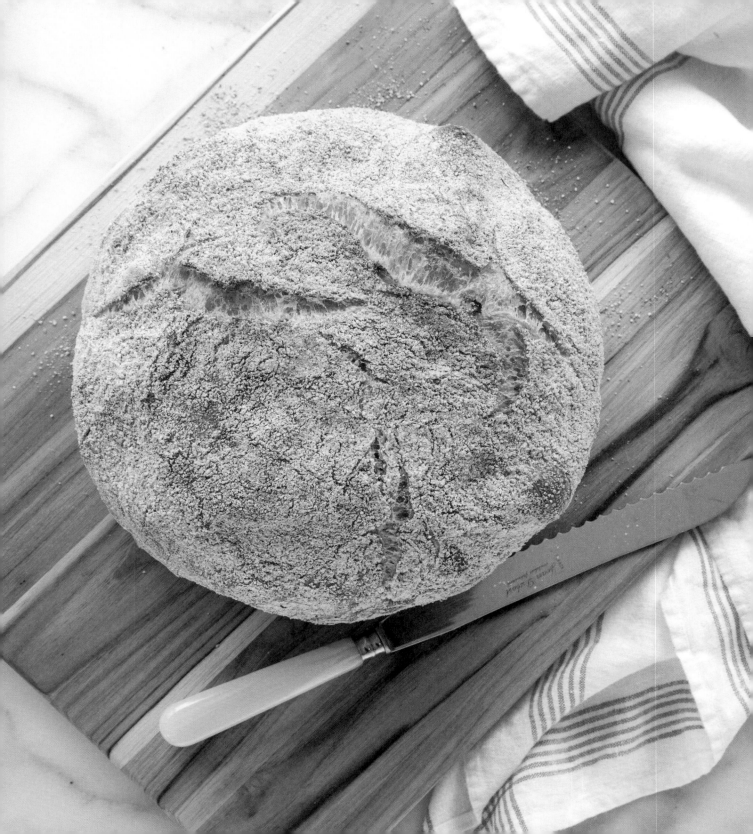

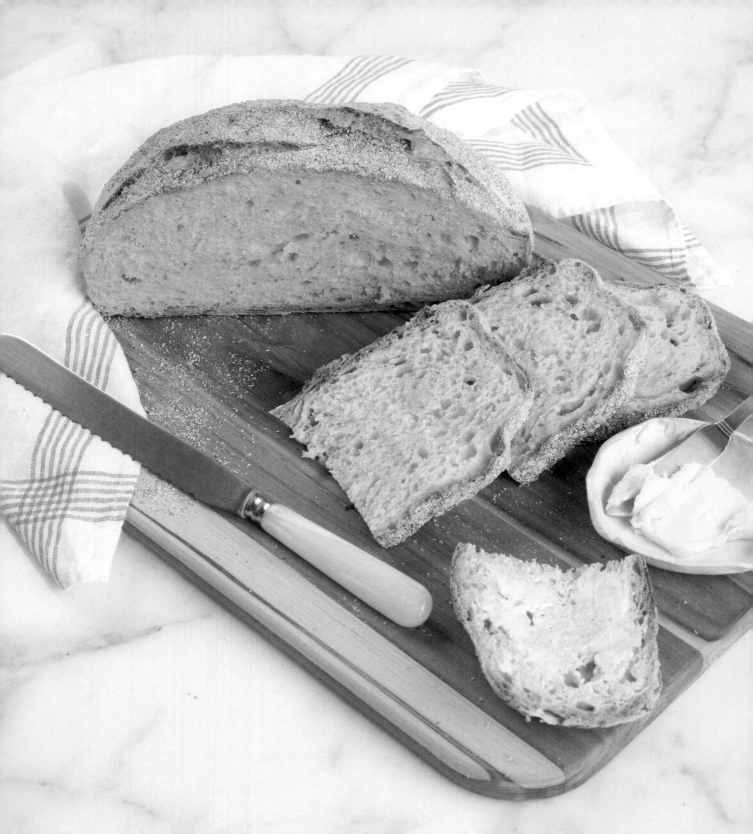

This recipe is adapted from the Sullivan Street Bakery's No-Knead Bread recipe, which appeared in The New York Times many years ago. I have come to find that bread is really a combination of art and science, and gauging what the bread needs to rise properly. The loaf will easily last for a whole week. Once it's baked and cooled, I usually put half in the freezer until I am ready to use it.

Beginner's Bread

Makes 1 loaf

2 teaspoons instant yeast

I teaspoon granulated sugar

2 1/2 cups lukewarm water
(I use half boiling water
and half cold tap water)

6 to 6 1/2 cups organic
all-purpose or bread flour
(or half white and half
whole-wheat flours)

2 teaspoons sea salt

Olives, walnuts, or cranberries
(optional)

I/4 to I/2 cup corn flour

1. In a small bowl, combine the yeast and sugar with 1/2 cup of the warm water. Let stand for 5 minutes until the mixture bubbles.

2. In a large bowl, combine 5 cups of the all-purpose flour and the salt. Add the remaining 2 cups warm water and the yeast mixture. Mix well.

3. Cover with plastic wrap and let stand in a warm place for at least 18 hours, until the surface gets bubbly.

4. Put the remaining 1 1/2 cups flour on a board. Turn the dough mixture out onto the board and sprinkle flour on top. Turn the dough mixture onto itself a few times until it is no longer sticky and let stand 15 minutes. (Note: if you are using one of the optional ingredients — olives, walnuts, cranberries — add it here.)

5. Coat a clean kitchen towel with corn flour. Knead the dough into a ball, turn it onto the kitchen towel, and wrap the towel around the it. Transfer to a medium bowl and let stand for 2 hours. The dough should roughly double in size.

6. Preheat the oven to 450°F. Thirty minutes before the dough is done rising, put a Pyrex bowl or cast-iron pot into the oven to warm. When the dough is ready, remove it from the towel and gently turn it into the pot.

7. Bake, covered, for 40 minutes. Uncover and bake 10 minutes longer, until the bread is nice and brown.

Congee or kicheree, is a rice porridge used frequently in Asia to soothe the stomach and ease digestion. It can be savory or sweet. Below are two possible additions for a sweet congee that makes a nice breakfast porridge.

Sweet Congee Two Ways

Serves 6 to 8

FOR THE CONGEE

1/2 cup short-grain brown rice

1/4 teaspoon sea salt

FOR THE POACHED QUINCE

3/4 cup maple sugar

1 cinnamon stick

4 slices fresh ginger, unpeeled

3 quince

Juice of 1 lemon

FOR THE STEWED FRUIT

1/4 cup pitted prunes

1/2 cup dried apples and/or apricots, halved

1/4 cup golden raisins

1 vanilla bean, split in half lengthwise

MAKE THE CONGEE

1. Put the rice, salt, and 5 cups of water in a large pot. Bring to a boil, reduce the heat to low, and simmer for 1 hour, stirring occasionally, until the rice has the thickened texture of porridge.

2. Add the poached quince and syrup (below) or the stewed fruit to the rice. Cook for another 10 minutes for flavors to infuse.

MAKE THE POACHED QUINCE

1. Combine 5 cups of water with the sugar, cinnamon, and ginger in a large pot. Bring to a boil.

2. Peel the quince and rub all over with lemon juice. Add to the pot.

3. Reduce the water to a simmer and cook the quince until just tender, 25 to 30 minutes (you don't want them to be too soft at this point because they will continue to cook after being added to the congee). Remove the quince from the pot, let cool, and cut into 1/2-inch cubes.

4. Meanwhile, raise the heat to high to boil the cooking liquid until reduced to a syrupy consistency. Add the poached quince and syrup to the congee.

MAKE THE STEWED FRUIT

1. Combine all the ingredients with 2 cups water in a small saucepan and bring to a boil.

2. Reduce the heat to low and let simmer until most of the liquid has boiled off, and the fruit is soft. Add the stewed fruit to the congee.

I tend to be more of a sweet scone fan but when I had some extra scapes in my fridge (and was tired of making the usual scape pesto), I decided to try using them in a savory scone. To my surprise, my whole family enjoyed them. They are best served warm with butter. (If you don't have scapes you can substitute minced garlic or chopped scallions.)

Gruyére & Garlic Scones

Makes 8 scones

1 tablespoon salted butter
    plus

1 stick chilled, salted butter, cut
    into small pieces

15 garlic scapes, thinly sliced
    (should yield about 1 cup)

1 cup Gruyère cheese,
    grated

2 cups plus 1 tablespoon
    organic all-purpose flour, plus
    more for flouring surface

1 tablespoon aluminum-free
    baking powder

1 teaspoon sea salt

3 large eggs

1/2 cup buttermilk

1. Preheat the oven to 400°F.

2. Melt 1 tablespoon butter in a small sauté pan and sauté the scapes until soft and lightly browned, 3 to 4 minutes. Let cool.

3. When cool, add the cheese and 1 tablespoon of the flour and mix well.

4. In a medium bowl, combine the 2 cups flour, the baking powder, and salt. Work in the remaining 1 stick butter with your fingertips until the mixture looks grainy.

5. In another small bowl, combine 2 of the eggs and the buttermilk.

6. Add the buttermilk mixture to the flour mixture and mix well. Then gently fold in the scape and cheese mixture. Mix until well combined.

7. Transfer to a floured board and knead lightly. Form the dough into a round approximately 1 inch thick and cut it into 8 wedges. Transfer to a baking sheet lined with Silpat or parchment.

8. In a small bowl, beat the remaining egg and brush on top of the scones. Bake for 20 to 25 minutes, until cooked through and a knife inserted in the center comes out clean.

This recipe is adapted from a dish I had at the Kripalu Center in Massachusetts. It's a delicious variation on traditional oatmeal, and it can even be prepared the night before. Greek yogurt makes an excellent accompaniment to these bars.

Baked Oatmeal Bars

Serves 4 to 6

1/2 cup unsalted butter, plus more for the pan

3 cups rolled oats

1 cup maple or date sugar

2 teaspoons ground cinnamon

2 teaspoons aluminum-free baking powder

1 teaspoon sea salt

1 cup almond* milk (you can also use cow's milk or any other alternative milk)

2 large eggs

2 teaspoons pure vanilla extract

3/4 cup dried cranberries or raisins

1/2 cup slivered almonds or walnuts

1. Preheat the oven to 350°F. Butter a 9x13-inch glass baking dish.

2. Melt the butter over medium-low heat in a small saucepan. Let it brown slightly but be careful not to let it burn.

3. In a large bowl, mix the oats, sugar, cinnamon, baking powder, and salt.

4. In a medium bowl, combine the milk, eggs, melted butter, and vanilla. Stir into the oat mixture and mix well.

5. Stir in the dried cranberries or raisins and almonds or walnuts.

6. Spread the mixture in the baking dish. Bake for 40 minutes, until the top is browned and a knife inserted in the center comes out clean.

*A NOTE ON ALMONDS: While I like almonds, I am mindful not to use them too much when cooking or baking because they require a lot of water to produce. In a world where water scarcity is a reality, I try to make food choices that do not worsen the problem.

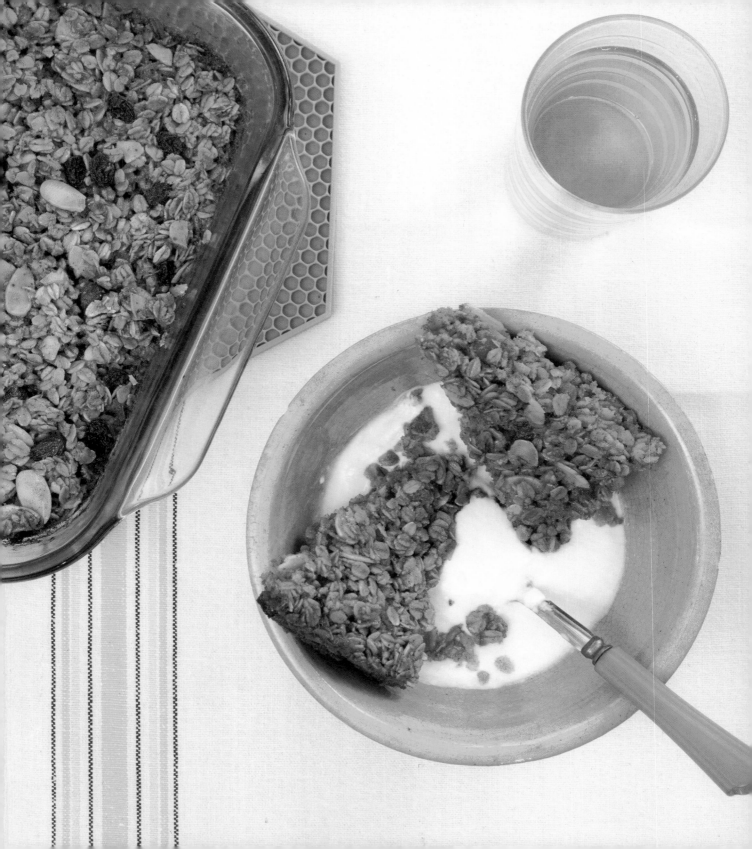

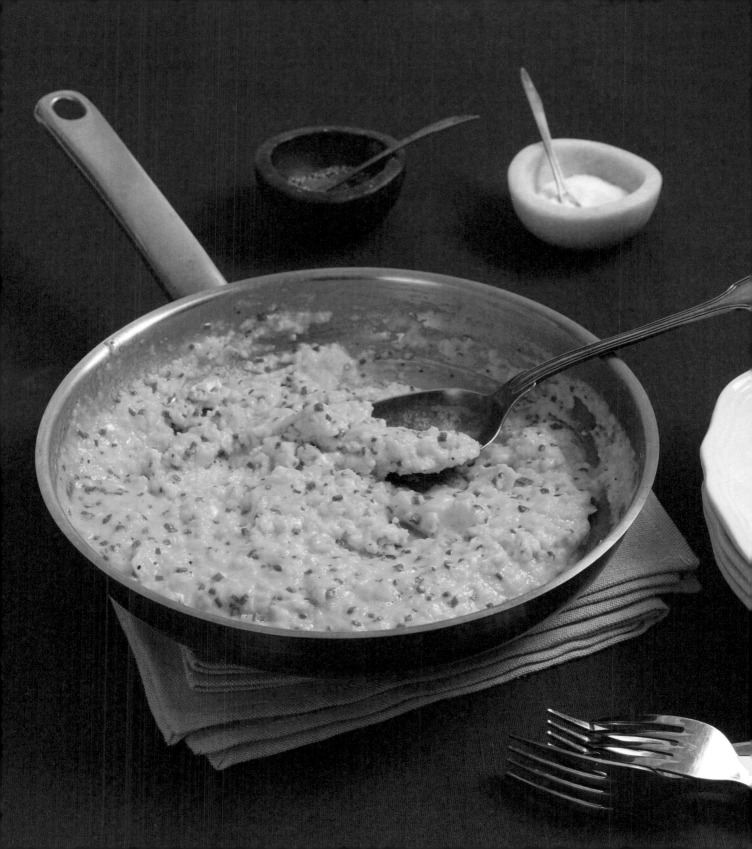

My husband and I have differing views about eggs. He feels that they can be eaten only for breakfast, while I think they're good anytime. I will happily eat a fried egg with salad for breakfast or dinner. Likewise, this recipe can be served for breakfast, brunch, or dinner, accompanied by a green or carrot salad.

Creamy Scrambled Eggs with Mascarpone & Chives

Serves 4 to 6

10 to 12 large eggs

3 tablespoons chopped fresh chives

4 to 6 tablespoons mascarpone cheese

1/2 teaspoon sea salt or, if you have it, black truffle salt

Freshly ground black pepper

4 tablespoons salted butter

1. In a large bowl, whisk the eggs until thoroughly combined. Add the chives and mascarpone and whisk until frothy. Add salt and pepper.

2. Melt the butter in a large sauté pan over medium heat. Add the egg mixture and whisk continuously while the eggs cook, 6 to 8 minutes, until just cooked through.

The Formula: **Frittata**

A frittata is essentially a quiche or tart without the crust, so you can use any of the fillings typically used for quiches to make a frittata. I find frittatas very versatile. They can be served for a formal brunch or lunch, or for a quick and easy dinner. They are also a good way to incorporate a variety of vegetables in one meal. **Serves 6**

1. Choose the vegetable combination (1 to 2 cups)

Select any that are in season, such as:

chopped scallions and spinach

shallots, peas, and thinly sliced asparagus

onions, sliced mushrooms, and diced red peppers

red onions and steamed broccoli florets

2. Choose the cheese (1 cup)

These are the ones I like to use:

grated Gruyère

crumbled feta

grated fontina

grated Cheddar

3. Choose fresh herbs or seasonings
(2 teaspoons, or to taste)

thyme leaves

chopped dill

sliced chives

crushed red pepper flakes

4. Plus basic ingredients

2 tablespoons butter or olive oil

sea salt and freshly ground black pepper

8 large eggs

5. Make the frittata

1. Preheat the oven to 350°F.

2. Mix the eggs with the cheese.

3. Melt 2 tablespoons of butter or olive oil over medium heat in a medium sauté pan. Add the type of onion you are using and sauté until soft, 3 minutes. Add the remaining vegetables and cook 3 to 5 minutes, until softened. Season with salt and pepper.

4. Reduce the heat and add the eggs and cheese. Using a metal spatula, gently lift the edges of the frittata so that the raw egg continuously flows to the bottom.

5. When the bottom of the frittata is mostly set, after about 7 minutes, put the pan in the oven.

6. Cook until the eggs are fully set and the top is browned, 15 to 20 minutes.

Kale & Red Onion Frittata, recipe on page 48 »

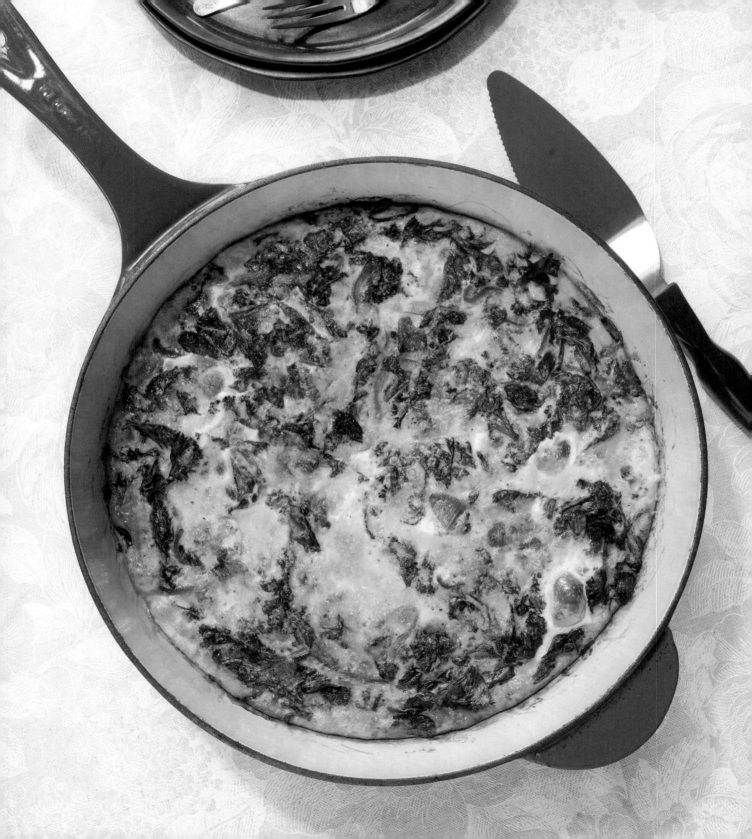

My family is fond of eggs, especially since two of us are vegetarians and eggs are a great source of protein. I am always looking for new and different ways to cook them and fresh ways to combine them with nutritious vegetables. You can easily substitute spinach or chard for the kale in this recipe. As with the Creamy Scrambled Eggs, this frittata can also be served for lunch or a light dinner.

Kale & Red Onion Frittata

(pictured on page 47)

Serves 6 to 8

2 tablespoons salted butter

1 medium red onion,
  thinly sliced

4 cups kale, stalks removed
  and leaves coarsely chopped

Sea salt

Freshly ground black pepper

8 large eggs, beaten

1 cup grated Gruyère cheese

1. Preheat the oven to 350°F.

2. Melt the butter over medium-low heat in a medium sauté pan. Add the onion and sauté until soft, 3 to 5 minutes. Add the kale and cook until wilted, about 3 minutes. Season with salt and pepper.

3. Combine the eggs and cheese in a medium bowl and mix.

4. Reduce the heat and add the eggs and cheese. Using a metal spatula, gently lift the edges of the frittata so that the raw egg continuously flows to the bottom.

5. When the bottom of the frittata is mostly set, after about 7 minutes, put the pan in the oven.

6. Cook until the eggs are fully set and the top is browned, 15 to 20 minutes.

Buckwheat is not actually a wheat grain; it is a cousin of rhubarb and therefore gluten-free. That said, buckwheat flour on its own works best for crêpes and pancakes. When it comes to tart or quiche doughs, you need to mix it with a wheat flour.

Buckwheat & Chard Tart

Makes one 10-inch tart

FOR THE CRUST

1 cup buckwheat flour

3/4 cup organic unbleached all-purpose flour, plus more for rolling

1/2 teaspoon sea salt

1/8 teaspoon aluminum-free baking powder

1/2 cup organic unsalted butter, chilled and cut into small pieces

3/4 to 1 cup ice water

FOR THE FILLING

2 tablespoons olive oil

1 medium red onion, thinly sliced

2 to 4 garlic scapes, thinly sliced, or 2 garlic cloves, finely chopped

1 large bunch chard, stemmed and leaves coarsely chopped

1/2 teaspoon crushed red pepper flakes

1 teaspoon sea salt

1/4 teaspoon freshly ground black pepper

5 large eggs

1 cup grated Gruyère cheese

MAKE THE CRUST

1. In a large bowl, combine the flours, salt, and baking powder and mix well. Add the butter and work it into the flour mixture with your fingertips until the mixture is crumbly. Gradually add the water and mix until the dough just comes together.

2. Gather the dough into a ball. Flatten it into a disk, wrap in plastic, and refrigerate for at least 1 hour.

3. Preheat the oven to 400°F. On a lightly floured surface, roll out the dough to fit a 10-inch fluted tart pan with a removable bottom. Carefully fit the dough in the pan and prick the bottom of the dough several times with a fork. Put a piece of parchment on top and fill with pie weights or dried beans.

4. Bake the crust for 15 minutes. Remove the weights and parchment and bake for an additional 10 minutes, until the edges of the tart are brown.

MAKE THE FILLING

1. Heat the oil in a large sauté pan. When hot, add the onion and garlic and sauté until soft. Add the chard and sauté until just wilted. Season with the red pepper flakes, salt, and pepper. Spread over the baked crust.

2. In a medium bowl, combine the eggs and 3/4 cup of the cheese and mix well. Pour over the chard.

3. Sprinkle the remaining 1/4 cup cheese on top and bake until the top is browned and the eggs are set in the center, 20 to 25 minutes. Remove the tart from the oven and let cool 5 to 10 minutes before serving.

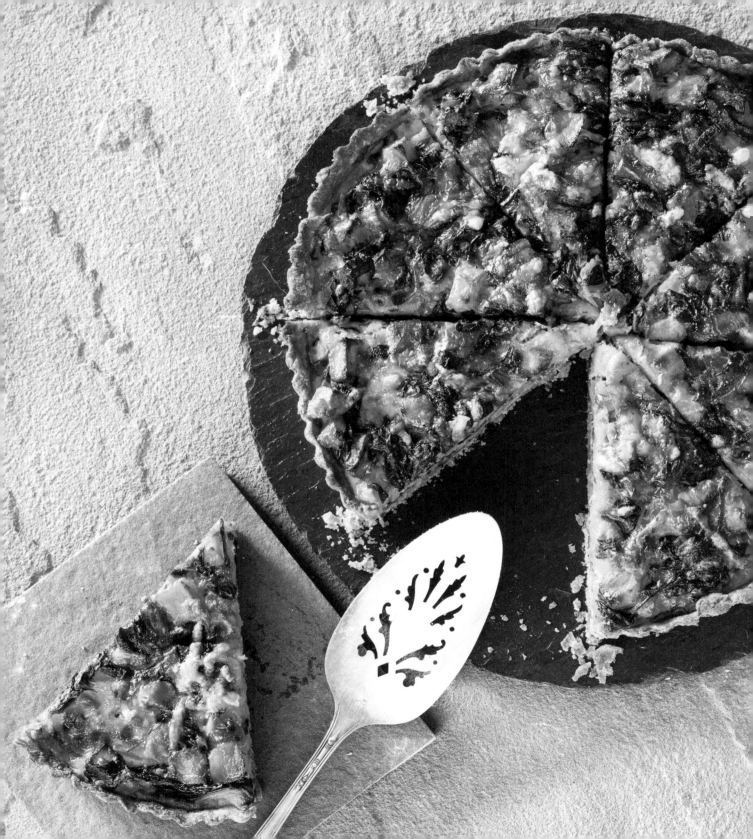

The great thing about tarts or quiches is that you can prepare all the ingredients ahead of time and then assemble everything at the last minute. Usually, I get the crust and filling ready the day before and add the eggs just before baking.

Spinach & Butternut Squash Tart

Makes one 10-inch tart

FOR THE CRUST

1 1/4 cups whole-wheat pastry flour (or half whole-wheat and half all-purpose), plus more for rolling

1/4 teaspoon sea salt

1/8 teaspoon aluminum-free baking powder

1/2 cup unsalted butter, chilled and cut into small pieces

1/4 cup ice water

FOR THE FILLING

3 cups 1/2-inch-cubed peeled butternut squash or other root vegetable of your choice

3 tablespoons olive oil

1 teaspoon sea salt, plus more to taste

Freshly ground black pepper

2 garlic cloves, chopped

1 medium onion, thinly sliced

5 ounces baby spinach

2 tablespoons balsamic vinegar

3 large eggs, lightly beaten

1 cup grated Italian Fontina cheese

MAKE THE CRUST

1. In a large bowl, combine the flour, salt, and baking powder and mix well. Add the butter and work it into the flour mixture with your fingertips until the mixture is crumbly. Gradually add the water and mix until the dough just comes together.

2. Gather the dough into a ball. Flatten it into a disk, wrap in plastic, and refrigerate for at least 1 hour.

3. Preheat the oven to 400°F. On a lightly floured surface, roll out the dough to fit a10-inch fluted tart pan with a removable bottom. Carefully fit the dough in the pan and prick the bottom of the dough several times with a fork. Put a piece of parchment on top and fill with pie weights or dried beans.

4. Bake the crust for 15 minutes. Remove the weights and parchment and bake for an additional 10 minutes, until the edges of the tart are brown.

MAKE THE FILLING

1. Preheat the oven to 400°F. On a large baking sheet, toss the squash with 2 tablespoons of the oil, 1/2 teaspoon of the salt, and the pepper. Roast for 20 to 25 minutes, until the squash is lightly browned and soft.

2. Heat the remaining 1 tablespoon of oil in a large skillet over medium heat and sauté the garlic until it browns lightly, about 30 seconds. Add the onion and sauté until soft, about 3 minutes. Add the spinach and a pinch of salt and sauté until wilted. Add the vinegar and transfer to a large bowl.

3. Stir the eggs into the onion and spinach mixture, then fold in the butternut squash and ¾ cup of the cheese. Season with salt and pepper to taste, and mix well. Pour the mixture into the prepared crust.

4. Sprinkle the remaining 1/4 cup cheese on top and bake until the filling is set, 25 to 30 minutes. Remove the tart from the oven and let cool 5 to 10 minutes before serving.

Grilled cheese sandwiches are a family favorite. They make it easy to accommodate vegetarians and non-vegetarians alike without too much extra effort. Accompanied by a soup, they make a hearty winter lunch.

Grilled Cheese Sandwiches

Makes 4 sandwiches

FOR THE CARAMELIZED ONIONS

1 tablespoon unsalted butter

1 tablespoon olive oil

1 medium onion, thinly sliced

FOR THE ROASTED SQUASH

1 squash, such as butternut or Delicata

2 tablespoons olive oil

Sea salt and freshly ground pepper, to taste

FOR THE SANDWICHES

8 slices white or whole-wheat bread

6 to 8 tablespoons salted butter, softened

Gruyère, Emmental, fontina or Cheddar cheese, sliced according to your preference

CARAMELIZE THE ONIONS

1. Melt the butter and oil in a large sauté pan over low heat.

2. Add the onion and cook over low heat, stirring frequently, until browned, 15 to 20 minutes.

ROAST THE SQUASH SLICES

1. Preheat the oven to 350°F.

2. Peel and thinly slice the squash (Delicata does not need to be peeled.)

4. On a large baking sheet, toss the squash with the oil and season with salt and pepper. Roast 20 to 25 minutes until the squash is lightly browned and soft.

MAKE THE SANDWICHES

1. Preheat the oven to 350°F.

2. Butter one side of each bread slice. Turn half of them over, lay the cheese slices on the unbuttered side of the bread and cover with the unbuttered side of the second slice.

3. If you are being adventurous, add the caramelized onions and roasted squash slices before covering the sandwiches with the second slices of bread.

4. Transfer the sandwiches to a baking sheet and bake for 10 to 15 minutes, until evenly browned, flipping them halfway through.

I love this dip because it has such an interesting combination of flavors but also because the warmth makes it comforting. You can serve this with a crudité platter, crackers, or on a sandwich accompanied by a handful of arugula.

Goat Cheese, Artichoke & Black Olive Dip

Serves 8 to 10

5 ounces artichoke hearts marinated in olive oil

1/2 cup fresh basil leaves

1/2 cup black olive tapenade (black olive paste)

1 garlic clove

1/2 cup grated Parmigiano-Reggiano

4 ounces fresh chèvre (goat cheese)

1/4 teaspoon sea salt

Freshly ground black pepper

1. Preheat the oven to 375°F.

2. Combine the artichokes, 1/4 cup of the oil they're packed in, the basil, tapenade, and garlic in a food processor or blender. Blend until smooth.

3. Transfer to a large bowl and fold in the cheeses, salt, and pepper.

4. Transfer to a baking dish, cover with foil, and bake until hot and bubbly, about 30 minutes.

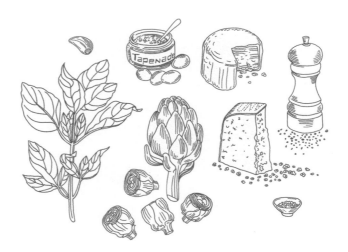

Whenever my kids are home from school on a snow or vacation day I am always
hard-pressed to come up with quick and nourishing lunch choices. Fortunately,
I usually have eggs and cheese in the fridge, which gives me two go-to options:
egg salad or grilled cheese sandwiches accompanied by mixed greens.

Egg Salad

Serves 6

8 to 10 hard-boiled eggs

1 large shallot, finely chopped

2 celery stalks, halved lengthwise
and thinly sliced

2 tablespoons drained and rinsed
capers, chopped

1/2 cup homemade (see below)
or store-bought organic
expeller-pressed mayonnaise,
more or less, to taste

1 1/2 teaspoons sea salt

Freshly ground black pepper

1/4 teaspoon paprika

1. Peel and finely chop the eggs.

2. In a large bowl, combine the eggs, shallots, celery, and capers.
Add the mayonnaise and mix well.

3. Season with salt, pepper, and paprika and mix well again.

*NOTE: If you have the time to make it — and it really
doesn't take that long — homemade mayonnaise is so much
better than store-bought. You can also flavor it with ingredients such as saffron and red chile powder and serve it
with steamed fish and an assortment of steamed vegetables,
which is one of my favorite traditional French dishes.

Homemade Mayonnaise

Makes 1 to 1 1/2 cups

1 garlic clove, peeled

Sea salt

1/2 teaspoon Dijon mustard

1 large egg yolk

Freshly ground black pepper

1 cup extra-virgin olive oil

1. In a large mortar, crush the garlic and salt with the pestle until
it becomes a smooth paste.

2. Transfer to a bowl and add the mustard, egg yolk, and pepper.
Mix well.

3. Slowly pour in the oil, a few drops at a time, whisking continuously
in the same direction until the mixture thickens to the consistency
of mayonnaise, 3 to 5 minutes. Season with salt and pepper.

*NOTE: If your mayonaise breaks and the
emulsion separates, add another egg yolk and
keep whisking until it comes back together.

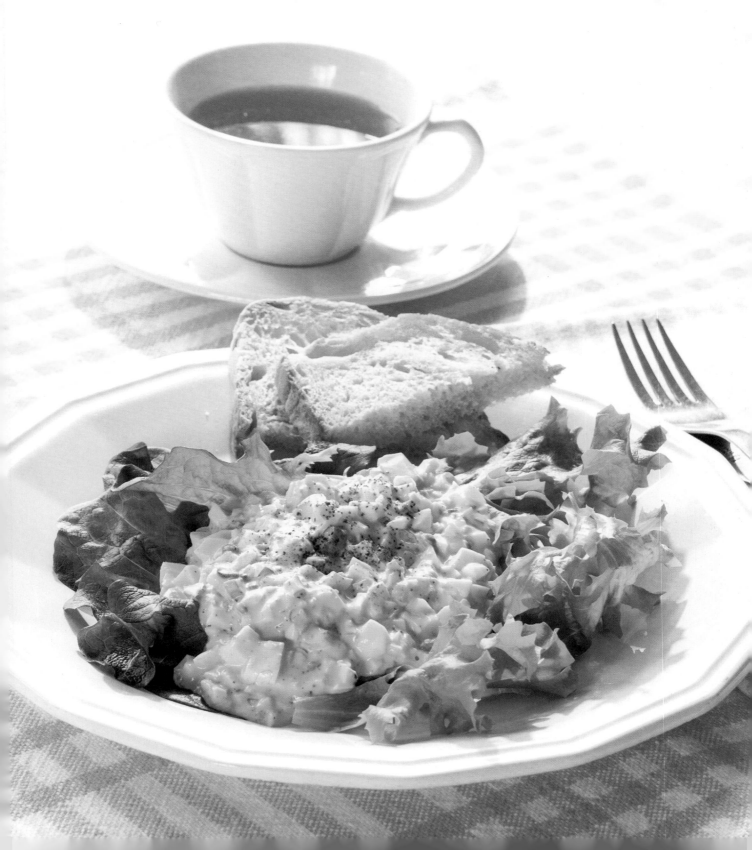

Soups

I wanted to have a special section for soups because they are so healthy. If the body's immune system is compromised in any way, soups are very healing because they have a lot of nutrients and are easy on the digestive system. I tend to prefer puréed soups to chunky ones, but any of these recipes can easily be made chunky if you prefer. The key to a good result is to use top-quality stock, preferably homemade.

Pea Shoot &
Asparagus Soup,
recipe on
page 70 »

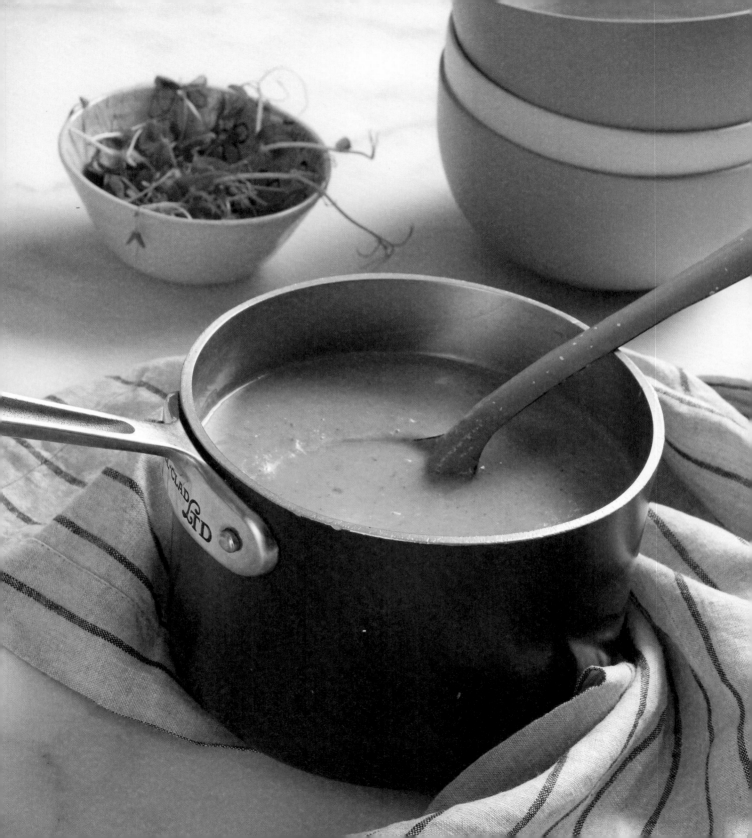

A good chicken or vegetable stock is an essential item to have in your kitchen. I usually make a large pot of stock and keep it in quart containers in the freezer so I always have some on hand when needed. To make vegetable stock, follow the chicken stock recipe and simply omit the chicken.

Chicken & Vegetable Stock

Makes 2 to 3 quarts

1 whole chicken, preferably free-range and organic

2 leeks, sliced

2 carrots, sliced

2 celery stalks, sliced

1 fennel bulb, quartered

1 large onion, halved

1 bouquet garni (2 bay leaves, 10 black peppercorns, 6 parsley sprigs, and 2 thyme sprigs wrapped together in a leek peel or cheesecloth)

1. Combine all the ingredients in a large pot. Add cold water to cover.

2. Bring to a boil and simmer for 1 hour, skimming froth from the surface when necessary and turning the chicken occasionally to ensure that it is fully cooked.

3. Let the stock cool slightly and then pour through a fine-mesh sieve into containers.

NOTE: The chicken can be reserved for chicken salad or chicken quesadillas, or added to any of the soups.

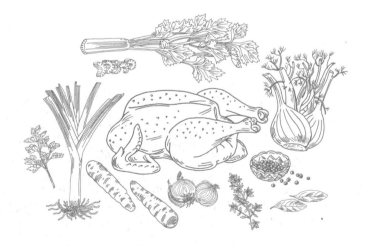

Towards the end of winter, when my family is fed up with eating root vegetables almost all the time, I find that the best way to use them yet again is to make soup. You can easily interchange the kohlrabi or turnip with rutabaga, celeriac, or potatoes. Served with some fresh bread, this soup makes a hearty lunch or a light dinner.

Kohlrabi, Turnip & Pea Soup

(pictured on page 61)

Serves 6

2 tablespoons salted butter

6 shallots, halved

6 small turnips, cleaned and quartered

4 medium kohlrabi, peeled and quartered

2 fresh thyme sprigs

6 to 8 cups chicken or vegetable stock

Sea salt

Freshly ground black pepper

1 pound frozen peas, thawed

1 cup coarsely chopped kale, chard, or spinach (optional)

1/4 cup crème fraîche (optional)

1. Melt the butter in a large pot over medium heat. Add the shallots, turnips, kohlrabi, and thyme. Sauté until the vegetables are very lightly browned.

2. Add stock to cover the vegetables and season with salt and pepper. Bring to a boil. Cover, reduce the heat to low, and simmer 20 to 25 minutes, stirring occasionally, until the vegetables are soft.

3. Add the peas and kale, chard, or spinach, if using, and cook an additional 2 to 3 minutes, until the peas are crisp-tender and the greens are wilted.

4. Let the soup cool, then purée using a hand-held blender or in a stand blender until smooth. Return the soup to the pot, reheat, and stir in the crème fraîche, if using.

The Formula: **Soup**

Soups are so easy to make and are a great source of nutrients and vitamins. And because they freeze so well, you can always have them on hand. Follow this basic formula to create your favorite new fundamental soups. **Serves 6 to 8**

1. Choose the fat (2 tablespoons)

salted butter

ghee

olive oil

2. Choose the allium
(1 to 2 cups chopped)

leeks

red or yellow onion

shallots

3. Choose the vegetable
(4 to 5 cups chopped)

Select any that are in season, such as:

leafy greens, including spinach, chard, and kale

root vegetables, including squash, carrot, and parsnip

asparagus and peas

4. Choose fresh herbs or seasonings (4 tablespoons)

chopped dill

grated fresh ginger and turmeric

sliced chives

5. Plus basic ingredients

4 to 6 cups of chicken or vegetable stock

heavy cream or crème fraîche

6. Make the soup

1. Heat the fat you have selected in a medium pot.

2. Sauté the allium in the fat until soft, 3 to 5 minutes.

3. Add the vegetables you choose and sauté lightly. If you decide to use potatoes to thicken the soup, you can add them here. Stir in herbs and/or seasonings.

4. Add chicken or vegetable stock to cover by about 1 inch (I recommend making your own — see the recipe on page 56 — but if you don't have any in your fridge or freezer, you can use water and a little white wine.

5. Bring to a boil, reduce the heat, cover, and cook until all the vegetables are soft. If you'd like to add cooked beans, you can add them here.

6. If you decide to purée the soup, remove it from the heat and let it cool before puréeing it with a hand-held immersion blender or in a stand blender.

7. Once off the heat, you can stir in heavy cream or crème fraîche to thicken the soup, if you like.

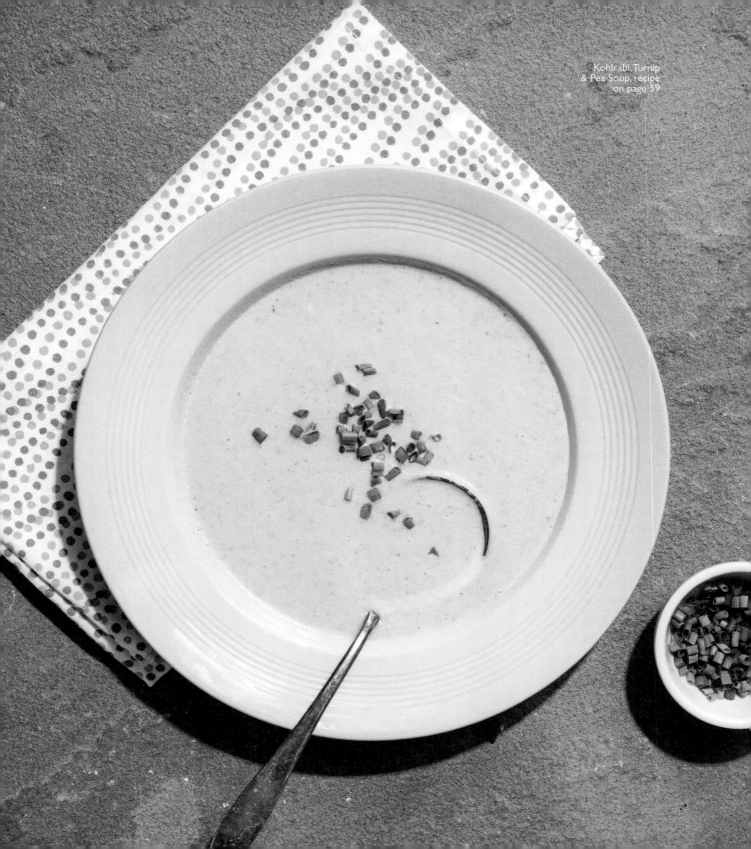

Kohlrabi, Turnip & Pea Soup, recipe on page 59

This is a hearty winter soup that is best served with fresh bread and butter. It's equally delicious with any variety of squashes or dark leafy green vegetables.

Red Lentil Soup with Butternut Squash & Kale

Serves 6

2 tablespoons ghee or butter

1 medium onion, coarsely chopped

4 garlic cloves, chopped

1-inch piece fresh ginger, peeled and grated

1 teaspoon ground turmeric

1 teaspoon roasted and ground cumin seeds

1 dried Indian red chile

2 cups dried red lentils

1 bay leaf

4 cups chicken or vegetable stock

2 cups large-cubed, peeled butternut squash or any other squash of your choice

1 pound kale, stalks removed and leaves thinly sliced

Sea salt

Freshly ground black pepper

1. Heat the ghee in a large pot over medium heat. Add the onion, garlic, ginger, turmeric, cumin, and chile. Sauté over medium-low heat until the onion is soft, about 5 minutes.

2. Add the lentils, bay leaf, stock, and 4 cups of water and bring to a simmer over medium-low heat. Cover and continue to simmer over low heat, stirring occasionally, until the lentils are fully cooked, about 30 minutes.

3. Add the squash and kale and simmer until the squash is soft, 15 to 20 minutes. Season with salt and pepper. Remove the soup from the heat and remove the bay leaf and chile.

4. Let the soup cool and then purée it using a hand-held immersion blender or in a stand blender until smooth. Return it to the pot and reheat before serving.

VARIATION:
Instead of adding the kale to the soup, you can make a kale pesto by combining the kale with 2 garlic cloves, 1/2 cup walnuts, 1/2 cup olive oil, 1 teaspoon sea salt, and 1/2 teaspoon freshly ground black pepper in a blender and puréeing to a smooth paste. Put a soupspoonful of pesto on top of the soup when serving.

This recipe is adapted from one an ayurvedic doctor gave my husband. Green mung beans are said to aid in the removal of toxins from the body and help to stimulate digestion.

Green Mung Bean Soup

Serves 6

1 cup sprouted green mung beans, soaked overnight, and drained

1 teaspoon ground turmeric

1/8 teaspoon asafetida powder*

2 bay leaves

2 curry leaves

2 tablespoons ghee or butter

1 teaspoon cumin seeds

1 teaspoon coriander seeds

1 teaspoon black mustard seeds

1 teaspoon fenugreek seeds

3 garlic cloves, thinly sliced

2 tablespoons fresh ginger, peeled and thinly sliced or chopped

1 teaspoon sea salt

Freshly ground black pepper

1. Combine the mung beans, 3 cups of water, the turmeric, asafetida, bay leaves, and curry leaves in a large pot. Bring to a boil over medium heat. Reduce the heat to low, cover, and let the soup simmer for 40 minutes, stirring occasionally, until the mung beans are soft.

2. While the soup is cooking, heat the ghee in a small sauté pan. Stir in the cumin, coriander, black mustard, and fenugreek seeds and let them sizzle for 30 seconds. Stir in the garlic and ginger and sauté until soft and lightly browned, 3 to 4 minutes. Remove from the heat.

3. Stir the spice mixture into the soup and season to taste with salt and pepper.

*NOTE: Asafetida powder is an Indian spice that can be found in most Indian grocery stores or online.

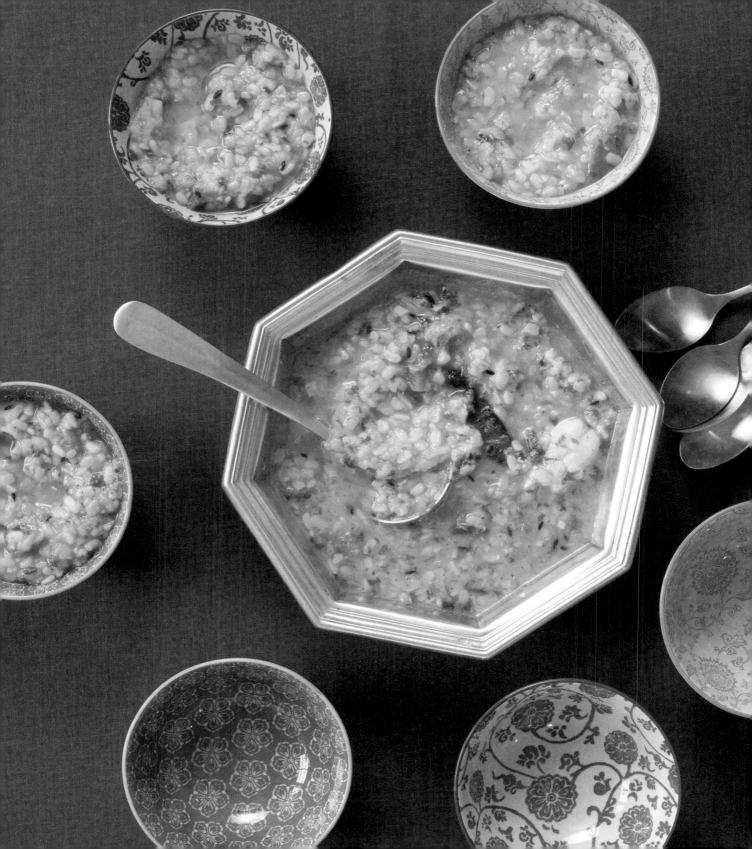

Dals are spiced lentil stews and they are very popular in India because they are so nourishing, can be served with a simple bowl of rice, and are super delicious. The wide variety of dals reflects the myriad cultures and cuisines in the country. Many families also have different ways of cooking dals, which is the case with this Khanna Dal. As the name suggests, this recipe is a big part of my husband's family's culinary tradition. Most dals use a "tarka" (or tempering), a mixture of spices fried in oil or ghee that serves to "lift" the flavors of the soup.

Khanna Dal

Serves 6

FOR THE DAL

I cup white urad dal beans*

1/2 cup yellow channa dal beans*

6 whole garlic cloves

I teaspoon ground turmeric

I teaspoon sea salt

FOR THE TARKA (tempering)

2 tablespoons ghee

Pinch of asafetida powder*
   (optional)

I teaspoon cumin seeds

I dried Indian red chile

I tomato, chopped

I tablespoon peeled and
   grated fresh ginger

2 tablespoons chopped
   fresh cilantro

MAKE THE DAL

1. Put the dals, garlic, turmeric, and salt in a medium pot, cover with water, and bring to a boil. Cook until the beans are soft but still firm, 30 to 45 minutes, skimming the froth from the top occasionally.

MAKE THE TARKA

1. Meanwhile, melt the ghee in a small frying pan. Add the asafetida, if using, then the cumin seeds. As soon as the cumin seeds begin to pop, add the chile, tomato, and ginger.

2. Fry everything until brown and aromatic. Remove from the heat and stir in the cilantro.

3. Stir the tarka into the dal and serve.

*NOTE: Dal beans and asafetida powder can
   be found in most Indian grocery stores or online.

It took me a while to learn to appreciate the nutty flavor of sunchokes (also called Jerusalem artichokes). Now, I grab them the minute they are available in farmers' markets. Though they lend themselves very easily to soups, they can also be sautéed, roasted, or made into a gratin. One thing to note is that sunchokes can be hard for some people to digest.

Sunchoke Soup

Serves 6

1 tablespoon fresh lemon juice

2 pounds sunchokes (also called Jerusalem artichokes)

4 tablespoons salted butter

2 leeks, white and light-green parts only, thinly sliced, then soaked in cold water to remove the grit

2 garlic cloves, chopped

8 cups chicken or vegetable stock

1/2 cup heavy cream (optional)

Sea salt

Freshly ground black pepper

1. Prepare a bowl of water large enough to hold the sunchokes. Add the lemon juice. Peel and quarter the sun chokes and put them in the water until ready to use.

2. Melt the butter in a large pot over medium heat. Add the leeks and garlic and sauté until soft, 8 to 10 minutes.

3. Drain the sunchokes and add them to the pot. Sauté for 5 minutes (see note; if using potatoes instead of heavy cream, add them now). Add the stock and bring to a boil. Reduce the heat to low, cover, and let the soup simmer until the sunchokes are soft, about 45 minutes.

4. Let the soup cool, then purée it using a hand-held immersion blender or in a stand blender until smooth. Return to the pot, reheat, and stir in the heavy cream, if using. Season with salt and pepper to taste.

NOTE: If you prefer not to use heavy cream, you can instead thicken the soup by adding 1 or 2 peeled boiling potatoes along with the sunchokes.

In my mind, cauliflower and sunchokes are a natural combination, similar to peas and carrots or asparagus and mushrooms. Combined, they lend this soup a richness that is very pleasing, especially in wintertime. If you can't find sunchokes, feel free to substitute artichoke hearts.

Curried Cauliflower-Sunchoke Soup

Serves 6

1 tablespoon fresh lemon juice

1 pound sunchokes (also called Jerusalem artichokes)

3 tablespoons salted butter

1 medium onion, thinly sliced

1 large head cauliflower (about 2 pounds), cut into medium-size florets

4 to 6 cups chicken or vegetable stock

1 teaspoon sea salt

Freshly ground black pepper

1 tablespoon curry powder, more to taste

1/4 cup crème fraîche (optional)

1. Prepare a bowl of water large enough to hold the sunchokes. Add the lemon juice. Peel and quarter the sunchokes and place them in the water until ready to use.

2. Melt the butter in a large pot over medium heat. Add the onion and sauté until soft, 8 to 10 minutes.

3. Drain the sunchokes and add them to the pot along with the cauliflower. Sauté until lightly browned.

4. Add the stock to cover and bring to a boil. Reduce the heat to low and simmer until the vegetables are soft, 30 to 40 minutes. Remove from the heat and season with salt, pepper, and curry powder.

5. Let the soup cool, then purée it using a hand-held immersion blender or in a stand blender until smooth. Return to the pot, reheat, and stir in the crème fraîche, if using.

Who doesn't love a good butternut squash soup in winter? Squash and ginger are another great warming and healing combination. Of course, the butternut squash can easily be interchanged with any other squash you would like to use, such as kabocha, honeynut, or buttercup.

Butternut Squash & Ginger Soup

Serves 6

3 tablespoons salted butter

I large onion, quartered

I garlic clove

I-inch piece fresh ginger, peeled

I butternut squash, peeled and coarsely cubed (you should have 6 to 8 cups of squash)

4 tart apples, peeled, cored, and coarsely chopped (gently toss with lemon juice to prevent browning)

Sea salt

Freshly ground black pepper

4 cups chicken or vegetable stock

1. Melt the butter in a large pot over medium heat. Add the onion, garlic, and ginger and cook, stirring occasionally, until the onion is soft, 2 to 3 minutes.

2. Stir the squash and apple pieces into the pot and sauté until lightly browned. Season with salt and pepper.

3. Pour in the stock and bring to a boil. Cover, reduce the heat to low, and simmer gently, stirring occasionally, until the squash and apples are very tender, about 40 minutes.

4. Let the soup cool, then purée it using a hand-held immersion blender or in a stand blender until smooth. Return the soup to the pot and reheat before serving.

Turmeric, a close cousin to ginger, is an anti-inflammatory and antioxidant root with a deliciously fragrant flavor. It is often found in Indian cuisine, and it is also used in traditional ayurveda to treat digestive issues, skin diseases, and cuts.

Carrot & Parsnip Soup with Turmeric & Ginger

Serves 6

2 tablespoons ghee or butter

2 leeks, white and light-green parts only, thinly sliced, then soaked in cold water to remove the grit

1 pound carrots, peeled and coarsely chopped

1 pound parsnips, peeled and coarsely chopped

1-inch piece fresh ginger, peeled

1-inch piece fresh turmeric, peeled

6 cups vegetable stock

1. Melt the ghee in a large pot over medium heat. Add the leek and sauté until soft, 3 to 5 minutes. Add the carrots, parsnips, ginger, and turmeric and sauté until the vegetables start to brown, an additional 2 to 3 minutes.

2. Pour in the stock and bring to a boil. Cover, reduce the heat to low, and simmer gently, stirring occasionally, until the vegetables are soft, 30 to 40 minutes.

3. Let the soup cool, then purée it using a hand-held immersion blender or in a stand blender until smooth. Return the soup to the pot and reheat before serving.

This is a lovely soup for springtime, wich can be served hot or cold. I like it with a dollop of crème fraîche on top. You can also garnish it with micro greens or some pretty edible flowers.

Pea Shoot & Asparagus Soup

Serves 6

3 tablespoons salted butter

1 medium onion, thinly sliced

2 medium Yukon Gold potatoes, peeled and quartered

1 bunch asparagus, trimmed and cut into 1-inch pieces

6 cups chicken or vegetable stock

1/2 pound pea shoots

Sea salt

Freshly ground black pepper

1/4 cup crème fraîche (optional)

Microgreens or edible flowers for garnish

1. Melt the butter in a large pot over medium heat. Add the onion and sauté until soft, 3 to 5 minutes.

2. Add the potatoes and asparagus and sauté for 2 to 3 minutes, until well coated with the butter.

3. Add the stock and bring to a boil. Cover, reduce the heat to low, and simmer until the potatoes and asparagus are soft, about 20 minutes.

4. Add the pea shoots and cook an additional 5 minutes, until just wilted. Season with salt and pepper to taste.

5. Let the soup cool, then purée it using a hand-held immersion blender or in a stand blender until smooth. Return it to the pot, reheat, and serve with a dollop of crème fraîche on top, if using, or garnish with microgreens or edible flowers.

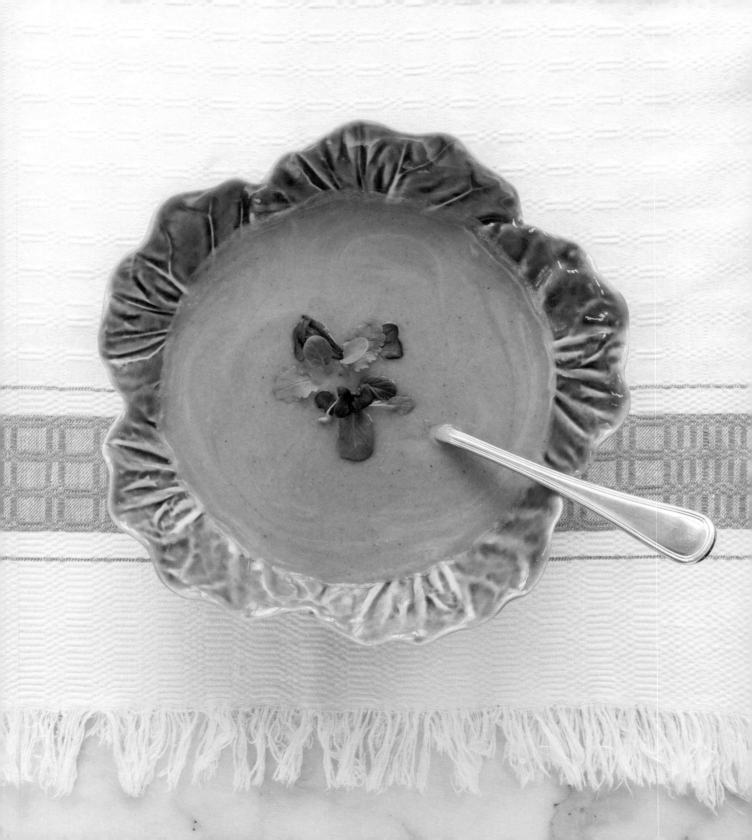

We don't typically think of soups for summer but this soup, which celebrates a trio of seasonal summer veggies, is delightfully refreshing on a hot summer evening. It can be served hot or cold. For a richer soup, add some cubed Cheddar cheese or feta.

Zucchini, Summer Squash & Corn Soup

Serves 6

3 tablespoons olive oil

1 medium onion, coarsely chopped

2 medium zucchini, coarsely chopped

2 medium summer squash, coarsely chopped

6 cups vegetable or chicken stock

3 ears of corn, kernels removed

2 to 3 dashes Tabasco sauce (optional)

Sea salt

Freshly ground black pepper

1. Heat the oil in a medium pot over medium heat. Add the onion, zucchini, and summer squash and sauté until soft and lightly browned, 5 to 7 minutes.

2. Add the stock and bring to a boil. Cover, reduce the heat to low, and simmer until the vegetables are soft, 10 to 15 minutes.

3. Add the corn and simmer another 5 to 10 minutes, until the kernels are soft. Add a few dashes of Tabasco, if using, and season with salt and pepper.

4. Let the soup cool, then purée it using a hand-held immersion blender or in a stand blender until smooth. Strain the soup through a fine-mesh sieve.

5. If serving cold, refrigerate for 2 to 3 hours, or until ready to serve.

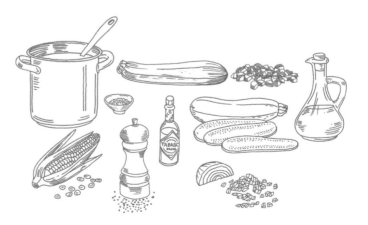

I like white beans because I find them lighter than other beans, making them a great choice when you want a soup that's filling but not too hearty. This white bean soup is fresh and colorful and can be served with crusty bread and a light green salad to round out a perfect summer's dinner.

Summery White Bean & Vegetable Soup

Serves 6 to 8

FOR THE BEANS
(4 cups cooled)

1 pound dried white beans

1 onion, quartered

1 bay leaf

1 sprig rosemary

FOR THE SOUP

4 tablespoons olive oil

2 cups chopped onion

2 cups diced carrots

2 cups diced fennel

2 cups 1-inch-chopped green beans

1 teaspoon chopped garlic

8 to 10 cups vegetable stock

2 cups frozen peas, thawed

4 tablespoons chopped fresh parsley

2 tablespoons chopped fresh mint

Pinch of crushed red pepper flakes

Grated zest of 1 lemon

Sea salt

Freshly ground black pepper

COOK THE BEANS

1. Put the beans in a pot with the onion, bay leaf, and rosemary. Cover with cold water. Bring to a boil, reduce the heat, and let cook until soft, 1 to 1 1/2 hours. Drain the beans and discard the onion, bay leaf, and rosemary.

MAKE THE SOUP

1. Heat the oil in a medium pot over medium heat. Add the onions, carrots, fennel, green beans, and garlic and sauté until the onions are translucent and the vegetables are softened, 5 to 10 minutes.

2. Add the stock and peas to the pot. Bring to a boil then reduce the heat and let simmer until the vegetables are soft, about 15 minutes.

3. Add the cooked white beans and simmer an additional 5 minutes.

4. Add the parsley, mint, red pepper flakes, and lemon zest. Mix well and season with salt and pepper.

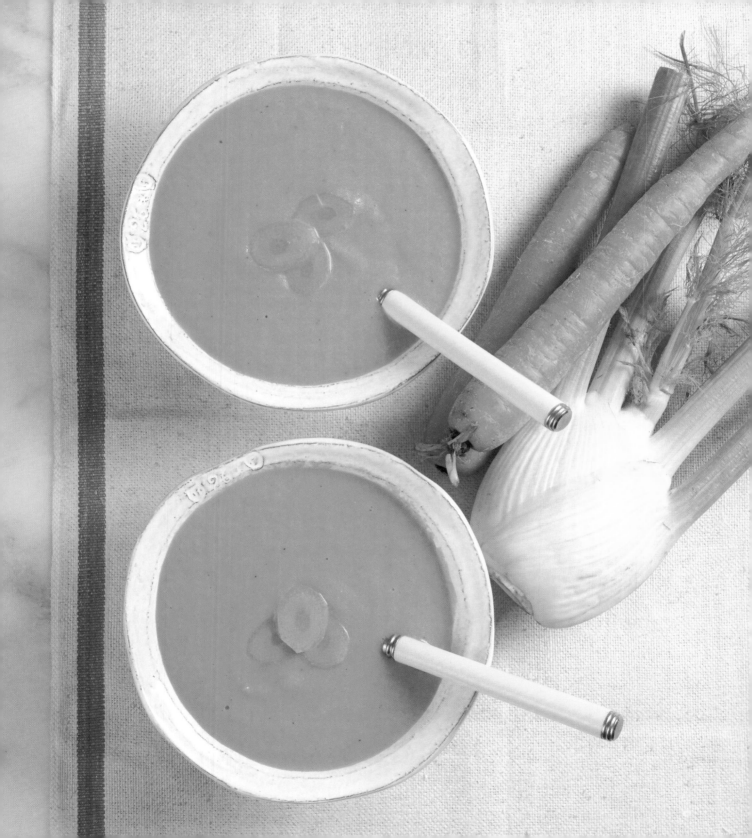

Carrots and fennel are another one of those natural pairings that everyone seems to love. This soup can also be served hot, but as a cold soup, it's pleasingly refreshing. I generally like to serve it with the Purslane Salad with Halloumi cheese (see page 92).

Chilled Carrot & Fennel Soup

Serves 6

2 to 3 tablespoons olive oil

1 medium onion, coarsely chopped

2 heads fennel, coarsely chopped, fronds reserved for garnish

6 carrots, peeled and coarsely chopped

6 cups vegetable or chicken stock

Sea salt

Freshly ground black pepper

Crème fraîche (optional)

1. Heat the oil in a medium pot over medium heat. Add the onions, fennel, and carrots and sauté until soft and lightly browned, 5 to 7 minutes.

2. Add the stock and bring to a boil. Cover, reduce the heat to low, and simmer until the vegetables are soft, 30 to 40 minutes. Season with salt and pepper.

3. Let the soup cool, then purée it using a hand-held immersion blender or in a stand blender until smooth. If serving cold, refrigerate the soup for at least 2 hours, until ready to serve.

4. Serve with a dollop of crème fraîche, if desired, and garnish with reserved fennel fronds.

Salads

When I was growing up, it was common to have salad after almost every meal because this is typical in Europe. It helps with digestion and cleanses the palate. This is a tradition I have continued with my family. It's a good way to incorporate nutrient-rich greens into our diet. When using cooked vegetables or grains, or thicker salad greens such as kale, romaine, or spinach, toss them with the salad dressing and let stand for 20 to 30 minutes before serving.

Mâche Salad with Shallots and Edible Flowers, recipe on page 88 (pictured here with Kale instead of Mâche) ››

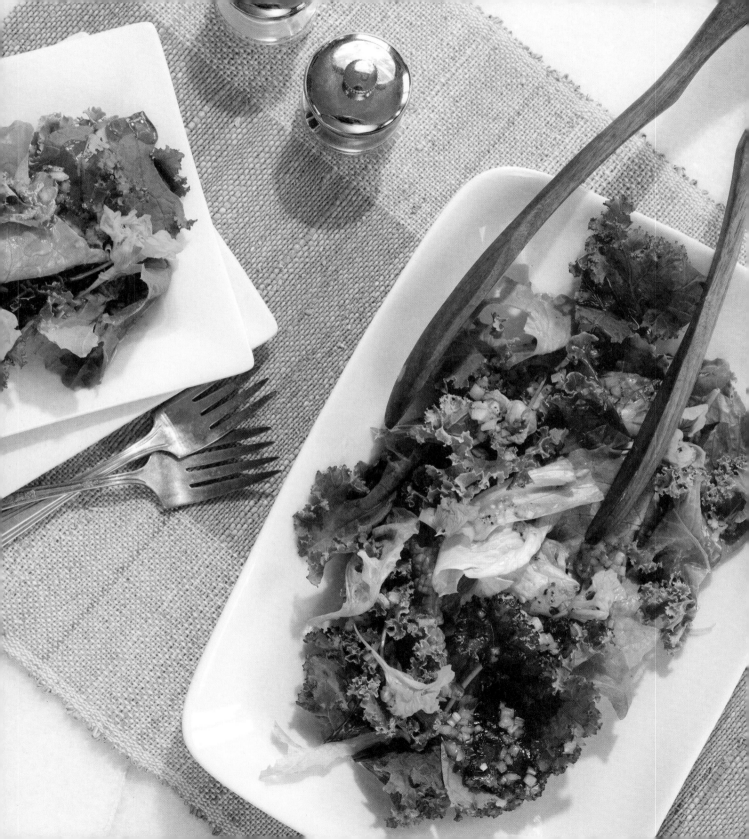

The Formula: **Vinaigrettes**

I use these four basic vinaigrettes for most of my salads. For more of my favorite dressings and vinaigrettes, take a look at the recipes for Grain Bowls on page 113. **Makes ½ to ¾ cup**

1. Choose a dressing

Apple-Cider Vinaigrette

2 tablespoons apple-cider vinegar

1/2 teaspoon Dijon mustard

1/2 teaspoon mayonnaise

1 garlic clove, grated

8 tablespoons extra-virgin olive oil

Sea salt

Freshly ground black pepper

Classic French Vinaigrette

2 tablespoons white wine vinegar

1/2 teaspoon Dijon mustard

8 tablespoons extra-virgin olive oil

Sea salt

Freshly ground black pepper

Garlicky Vinaigrette

2 tablespoons white-wine vinegar

1/2 teaspoon Dijon mustard

1 garlic clove, grated

8 tablespoons extra-virgin olive oil

Sea salt

Freshly ground black pepper

Shallot Vinaigrette

2 tablespoons Champagne vinegar

1/2 teaspoon honey

1 small shallot, finely chopped

6 tablespoons extra-virgin olive oil

Sea salt

Freshly ground black pepper

2. Make the dressing

1. In a small bowl, whisk all the ingredients except the oil.

2. Add the oil, 1 tablespoon at a time, whisking continuously until the dressing is well mixed. If you are using mayonnaise or mustard, whisk until the dressing is fully emulsified.

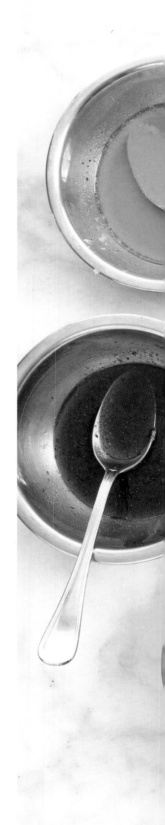

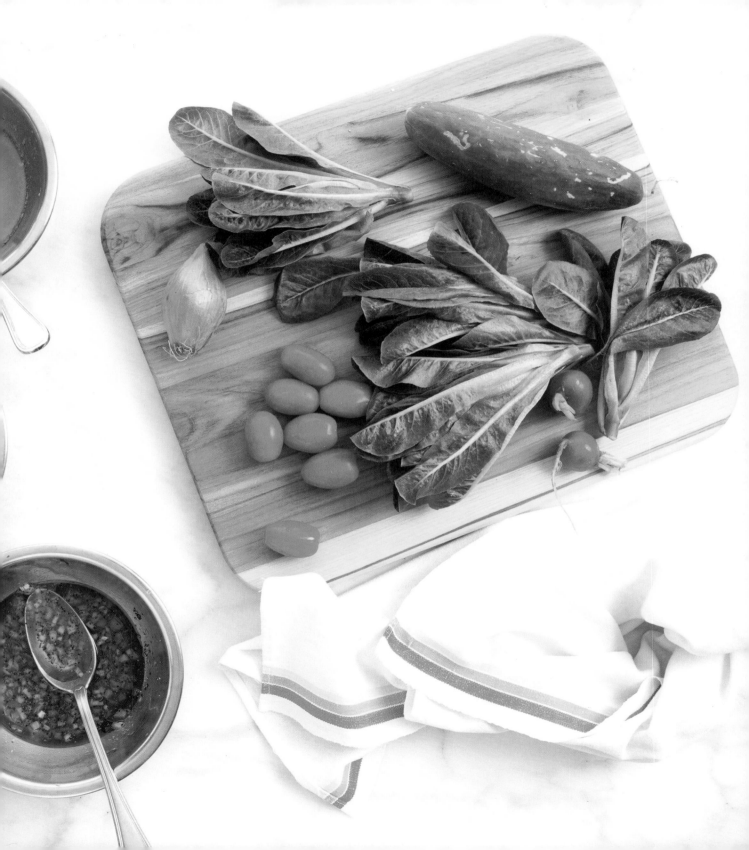

I love to use baby kale in salads because it is not as thick and chewy as mature kale. Also, mature leafy greens like spinach, kale, chard, and beet greens contain a lot of oxalic acid, which can prevent the absorption of important vitamins and minerals like calcium and iron. When these greens are cooked, the oxalic acid is broken down.

Baby Kale Caesar Salad

Serves 4 to 6

FOR THE DRESSING

2 garlic cloves, grated

1/4 cup fresh lemon juice

2 anchovy fillets packed in oil (optional, but they are a good source of protein and Omega 3 fatty acids)

Sea salt (if using anchovies, you will probably need very little salt)

Freshly ground black pepper

1/2 cup extra-virgin olive oil

FOR THE SALAD

3 to 4 slices whole-wheat or spelt bread, cut into 1/2-inch cubes

1/4 cup extra-virgin olive oil

6 to 8 cups baby kale

1/2 cup thinly sliced Parmigiano-Reggiano (I like to use a vegetable peeler to slice the cheese)

MAKE THE DRESSING

1. In a small bowl, whisk all the dressing ingredients except the oil. If using the anchovies, mix until the fillets have dissolved into the dressing, 1 to 2 minutes.

2. Add the oil, 1 tablespoon at a time, whisking continuously until the dressing is well mixed.

MAKE THE SALAD

1. Preheat the oven to 350°F.

2. Toss the bread cubes and the oil on a rimmed baking sheet until the cubes are well coated. Bake for 15 to 20 minutes, stirring halfway through, until brown and crisp.

3. In a large bowl, combine the kale and croutons. Add the dressing and toss well. Add half of the cheese and mix again. Top with the remaining cheese.

This salad is kind of like a kale slaw. You can interchange any leafy green, such as spinach or chard, for the kale and add thinly sliced red onions for a bit of a kick. For the tastiest results toss the dressing with the ingredients 20 to 30 minutes before serving so it can be fully absorbed.

Kale with Cabbage & Carrots

Serves 6 to 8

FOR THE DRESSING

Juice of 1 lemon

1 garlic clove, grated

1 small shallot, finely chopped

1 teaspoon Dijon mustard

Sea salt

Freshly ground black pepper

8 tablespoons extra-virgin
   olive oil

FOR THE SALAD

1 bunch kale, stalks removed
   and leaves thinly sliced

1 red bell pepper, ribs and seeds
   removed and pepper thinly sliced

1 yellow bell pepper, ribs and seeds
   removed and pepper thinly sliced

2 to 3 cups thinly sliced
   red cabbage

2 to 3 carrots, shredded

MAKE THE DRESSING

1. In a small bowl, whisk the dressing ingredients, except for the oil.

2. Add the oil, 1 tablespoon at a time, whisking continuously until the dressing is well mixed.

MAKE THE SALAD

1. In a large bowl, combine the salad ingredients. Add the dressing and toss well.

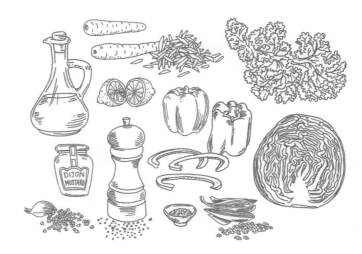

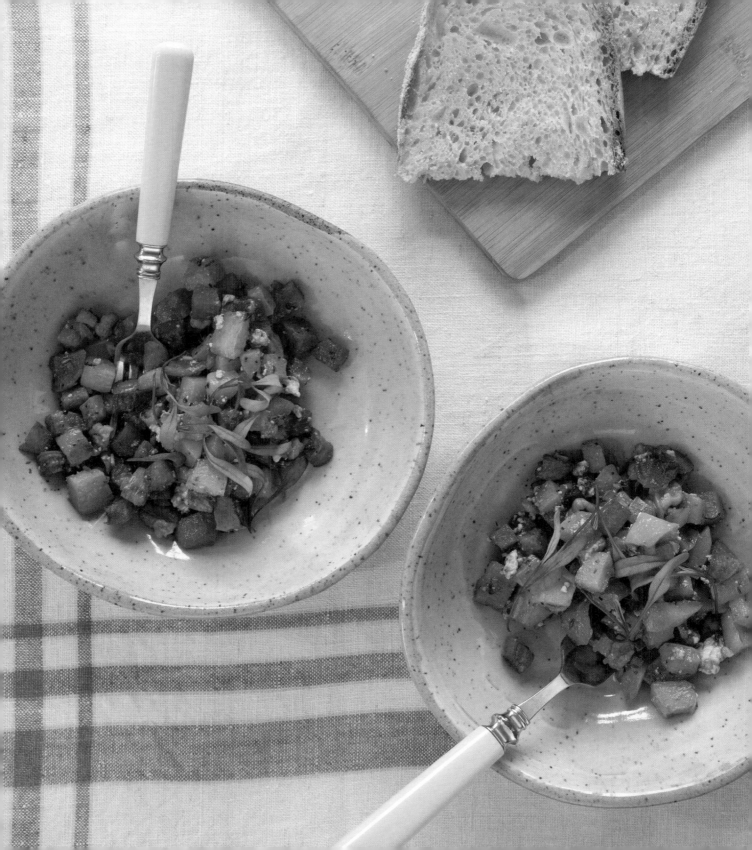

This hearty salad could easily be made with parsnips and sweet potatoes, or using leftover roasted vegetables. Served with quinoa or barley, it becomes a substantial meal. When we have people over for lunch, I serve this colorful dish with a quiche or frittata.

Beet & Butternut Squash Salad with Feta Cheese

Serves 6 to 8

FOR THE DRESSING

2 tablespoons balsamic vinegar

1 teaspoon Dijon mustard

Sea salt

Freshly ground black pepper

8 tablespoons extra-virgin
olive oil

FOR THE SALAD

4 medium-to-large beets, peeled
and cut into 1/2-inch cubes

1 small butternut squash, peeled
and cut into 1/2-inch cubes

2 tablespoons extra-virgin
olive oil

Sea salt

Freshly ground black pepper
to taste

1/2 to 3/4 cup crumbled feta cheese

1/4 cup coarsely chopped walnuts

2 tablespoons fresh thyme leaves

MAKE THE DRESSING

1. In a small bowl, whisk the dressing ingredients, except for the oil.

2. Add the oil, 1 tablespoon at a time, whisking continuously until the dressing is well mixed.

MAKE THE SALAD

1. Heat the oven to 400°F.

2. Toss the beets and squash on a rimmed baking sheet with the oil, salt, and pepper and roast, stirring halfway through, until tender and lightly browned, about 20 minutes. Remove from the oven and let cool completely.

3. In a large bowl, combine the beets, squash, feta, walnuts, and thyme.

4. Toss with the dressing and let the salad sit for 10 to 15 minutes before serving.

I normally make this salad with mesclun or arugula, but when I tried it with radicchio, it was a big hit. The radicchio and blue cheese are offset by the pear and cranberries, so it's a nice combination of spicy and sweet.

Winter Radicchio & Frisée Salad

Serves 6

FOR THE DRESSING

2 tablespoons white wine vinegar

1/2 teaspoon Dijon mustard

Sea salt

Freshly ground black pepper

6 to 8 tablespoons extra-virgin olive oil

FOR THE SALAD

1 head of radicchio, sliced

1 head of frisée lettuce, sliced

2 medium Bosc or Anjou pears, peeled, cored, and sliced into thin wedges

1/4 cup crumbled blue cheese (I like to use Roquefort, but any local blue cheese will do)

1/4 cup coarsely chopped walnuts

1/4 cup dried cranberries

MAKE THE DRESSING

1. In a small bowl, whisk all the dressing ingredients except the oil.

2. Add the oil, 1 tablespoon at a time, whisking continuously until the dressing is well-mixed.

MAKE THE SALAD

1. In a large bowl, combine the salad ingredients. Add the dressing and toss well.

A chance discovery of purple Brussels sprouts and purple cauliflower at my local market inspired me to make a shaved Brussels sprout and cauliflower salad. Of course, this tastes just as good with the more common green and white varieties.

Shaved Purple Brussels Sprout & Purple Cauliflower Salad

Serves 6 to 8

FOR THE DRESSING

2 tablespoons apple-cider vinegar

I teaspoon mustard

I teaspoon mayonnaise

I garlic clove, grated

Sea salt

Freshly ground black pepper

8 tablespoons extra-virgin olive oil

FOR THE SALAD

Sea salt

I small-to-medium head of cauliflower, cut into bite-size pieces

I pound Brussels sprouts, trimmed, and thinly sliced or shredded using a food processor

1/2 cup Pecorino Romano cheese, peeled into thin strips with a vegetable peeler

1/2 cup coarsely chopped walnuts

MAKE THE DRESSING

1. In a small bowl, whisk all the dressing ingredients, except the oil.

2. Add the oil, 1 tablespoon at a time, whisking continuously until the dressing is well-mixed.

MAKE THE SALAD

1. Bring a large pot of salted water to a boil. Add the cauliflower and boil for 2 to 3 minutes, or until just tender. Drain and put in a serving bowl.

2. Add the Brussels sprouts, cheese, and walnuts to the bowl.

3. Toss with the dressing and let the salad sit for 10 to 15 minutes before serving.

A friend of mine once made this for dinner on a summer evening, and it quickly became one of my favorite summer salads. I would recommend serving it with some grilled fish, chicken, or tempeh.

Broccoli, Green Bean & Cherry Tomato Salad

Serves 6 to 8

Sea salt

2 pounds broccoli, cut into bite-size pieces, about 1 inch wide (including some stem)

1 pound green beans, trimmed and cut into 1 1/2-inch pieces

2 quarts cherry or grape tomatoes, halved

Large pinch of crushed red pepper flakes

3 to 4 tablespoons extra-virgin olive oil, more as desired

Freshly ground black pepper

1. Bring a large pot of salted water to a boil. Meanwhile, prepare a large bowl of ice water. Blanch the broccoli for 5 to 6 minutes, until just tender. Transfer the broccoli to the ice water, reserving the boiling water.

2. Return the water in the pot to a boil if necessary. Blanch the green beans until just tender, 4 to 5 minutes. Transfer the green beans to the ice water.

3. Once the broccoli and green beans are cool, dry them on paper towels and transfer to a large salad bowl.

4. Add the tomatoes, red pepper flakes, oil, salt, and pepper.

5. Let the salad sit for 20 minutes before serving.

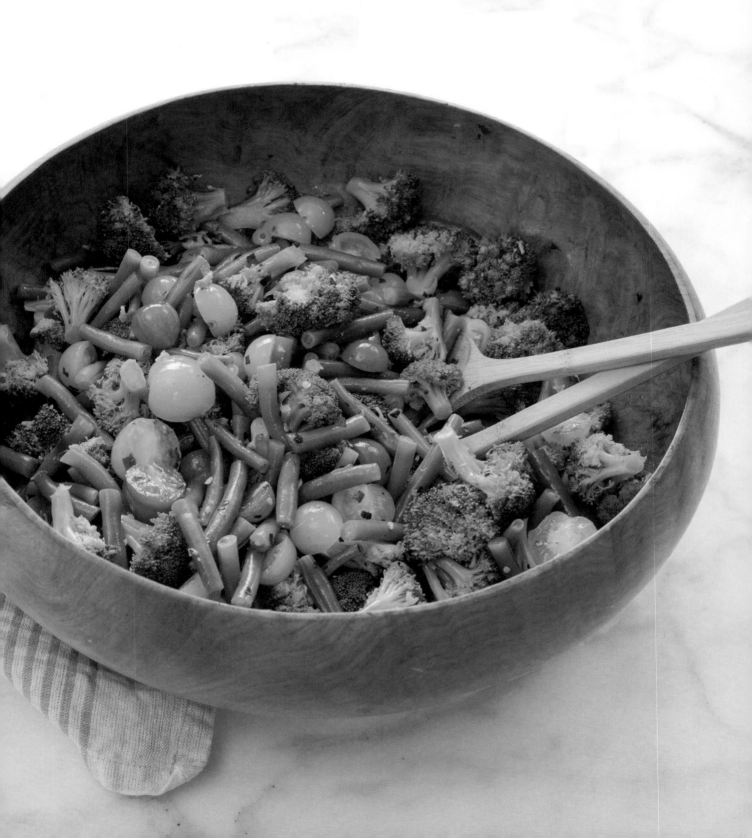

I also make this salad with baby kale (pictured on page 77) or any other delicate leafy green. When we have people over for dinner, this pretty dish never fails to impress. Alternatively, you can serve it with a fried egg on top for a sophisticated lunch main.

Mâche Salad with Shallots & Edible Flowers

(pictured with kale on page 77)

Serves 6

FOR THE DRESSING

2 tablespoons Champagne vinegar

1 large or 2 small shallots, finely chopped

Sea salt

Freshly ground black pepper

6 tablespoons extra-virgin olive oil

FOR THE SALAD

6 to 8 cups mâche greens or baby kale

Handful of edible flowers, such as nasturtiums or pansies

MAKE THE DRESSING

1. In a small bowl, whisk all the dressing ingredients except the oil.

2. Add the oil, 1 tablespoon at a time, whisking continuously until the dressing is well mixed.

MAKE THE SALAD

1. In a large bowl, combine the salad ingredients. Add the dressing and toss well.

At the end of winter, I couldn't decide what to do with the kohlrabi, red cabbage, and turnips that were sitting in my fridge, and my children had reached their limit of roasted root vegetables. This salad solved both problems—it's fresh, crisp, and has a little kick to it.

Kohlrabi, Red Cabbage, Turnip & Carrot Slaw

Serves 6 to 8

FOR THE DRESSING

4 tablespoons mayonnaise

2 tablespoons apple-cider vinegar

1 tablespoon Dijon mustard

1/2 teaspoon honey

Sea salt

Freshly ground black pepper

FOR THE SALAD

1 large or 2 small kohlrabi, peeled and shredded

1/4 head of red cabbage, cored and shredded

3 to 4 turnips, peeled and shredded

4 to 6 carrots, peeled and shredded

MAKE THE DRESSING

1. In a small bowl, whisk all the dressing ingredients until fully emulsified.

MAKE THE SALAD

1. In a large bowl, combine the salad ingredients and toss with the dressing. Let the salad sit for 20 minutes before serving.

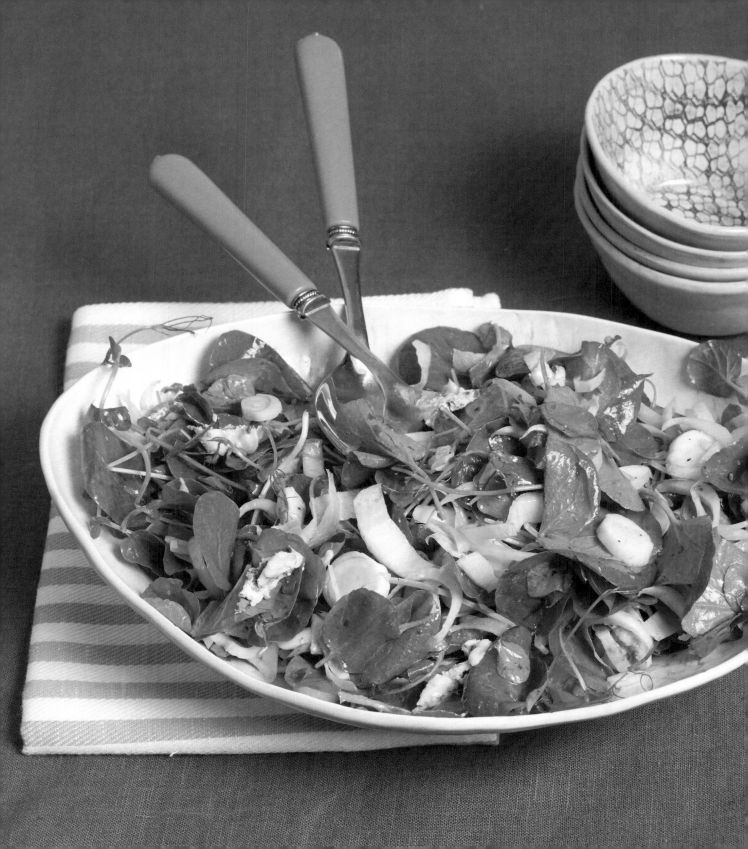

My family loves endive salad with Roquefort cheese. One day, I decided to add pea shoots and watercress for a little green, and I really liked the result. The Roquefort adds a rich creaminess to the bitter greens. You can also add thinly sliced Radicchio for a touch of color.

Pea Shoot, Watercress & Endive Salad with Roquefort

Serves 6

FOR THE DRESSING

2 tablespoons white-wine vinegar

1 teaspoon Dijon mustard

Sea salt

Freshly ground black pepper

6 to 8 tablespoons extra-virgin olive oil

FOR THE SALAD

3 to 4 ounces pea shoots

1 bunch watercress, leaves trimmed and stems removed

2 medium endives, trimmed and thinly sliced crosswise

1/4 cup crumbled Roquefort

MAKE THE DRESSING

1. In a small bowl, whisk all the dressing ingredients except the oil.

2. Add the oil, 1 tablespoon at a time, whisking continuously until the dressing is well mixed.

MAKE THE SALAD

1. In a large bowl, combine the salad ingredients and toss with the dressing. Let the salad sit for 5 to 10 minutes before serving.

Purslane is a weed native to India and Persia. But it's probably also growing somewhere in your garden. Though only a humble weed, it happens to be rich in vitamins, minerals, and Omega-3 fatty acids.

Purslane Salad with Halloumi Cheese

Serves 6 to 8

FOR THE DRESSING

2 tablespoons red-wine vinegar

I small shallot, finely chopped

I teaspoon dried oregano

Sea salt

Freshly ground black pepper

8 tablespoons extra-virgin
    olive oil

FOR THE SALAD

8 ounces halloumi cheese (you can
    also use feta cheese if you prefer)

2 tablespoons extra-virgin olive oil

I pound purslane leaves and tender
    sprigs

I red bell pepper, ribs and seeds
    removed and pepper thinly sliced

I yellow bell pepper, ribs and seeds
    removed and pepper thinly sliced

I pint cherry tomatoes, halved

I cucumber, peeled and thinly
    sliced into rounds

I/4 cup pitted green olives

MAKE THE DRESSING

1. In a small bowl, whisk all the dressing ingredients except the oil.

2. Add the oil, 1 tablespoon at a time, whisking continuously until the dressing is well mixed.

MAKE THE SALAD

1. Cut the cheese into 1/4-inch-thick slices. Heat the oil in a small sauté pan over medium heat and cook the cheese until golden brown, 3 to 4 minutes per side. Remove from the heat, let cool, and cut into wedges.

2. In a large bowl, combine the cheese with the remaining salad ingredients and toss with the dressing.

3. Let the salad sit for 20 to 30 minutes before serving.

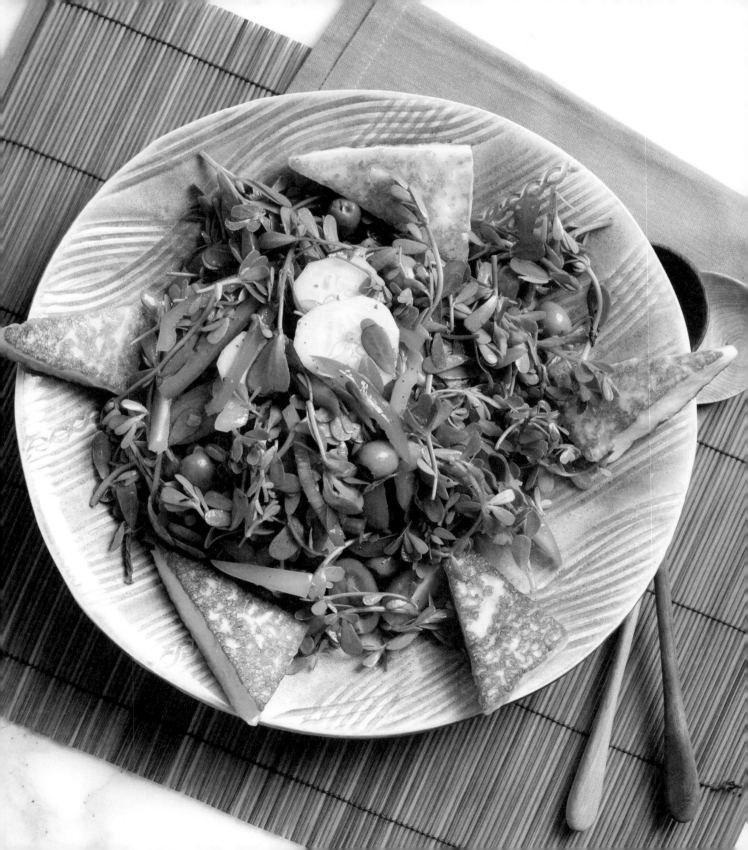

Entrées

In my household, we generally eat vegetarian three or four days a week, and eat meat, poultry, or fish the remainder of the days. With that balance in mind, these entrée recipes are designed to incorporate lots of fresh vegetables and whole grains in your diet. I've also included a few recipes featuring meat, poultry, and fish, but you'll find that even they are complemented with plenty of vegetables and healthy whole grains.

Steamed Arctic Char with Sautéed Leeks & Mushrooms, recipe on page 97 »

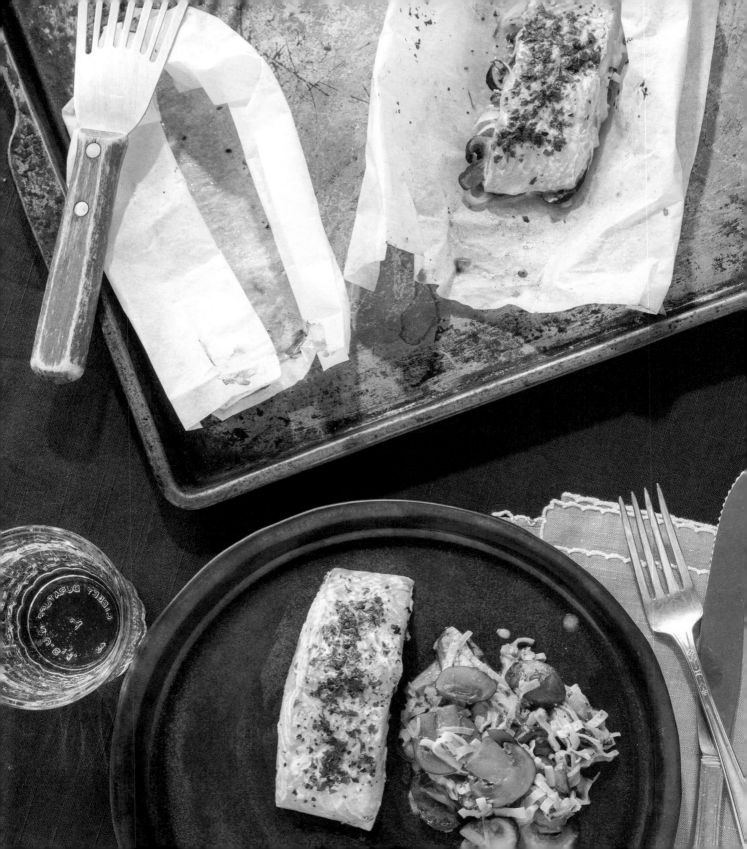

The Formula: **Fish en Papillote with Vegetables**

I love to steam fish in parchment paper because it's easy and mess-free but also because the fish retains its inherent moisture. When accompanied by an assortment of steamed or sautéed vegetables, it makes a light but nourishing dish. **Serves 6**

1. **Choose the fish** (about six 5-ounce fillets)

Select thick, firm-fleshed fish which won't flake when cooked, such as:

halibut

arctic char

wild salmon

2. **Choose the vegetable combination** (about 2 cups)

chopped shallots and thinly sliced fennel

julienned carrots and/or parsnips

sliced carrots with snap peas or snow peas

3. **Choose the herbs** (1/4 cup)

flat-leaf parsley

dill

chives

4. **Plus basic ingredients for the packages**:

6 tablespoons salted butter, softened

6 tablespoons white wine

sea salt and freshly ground black pepper

5. **Make the fish**

1. Preheat the oven to 350°F.

2. Cut 6 pieces of parchment paper large enough to enclose each fish fillet.

3. Place some of the vegetables on each piece of parchment. Add 1/2 tablespoon softened butter and 1 tablespoon of wine to each packet. Season with salt and pepper.

4. Place a piece of fish on top of the vegetables in each packet and season with salt and pepper. Rub 1/2 tablespoon of softened butter onto each piece of fish.

5. Sprinkle the herbs over the fish and vegetables. Wrap each packet with the parchment paper so that fish and vegetables are fully enclosed.

6. Bake the packets for 15 to 25 minutes, until the fish is fully cooked (cooking time will vary depending on the type and thickness of the fish: Wild salmon and arctic char will take less time than halibut).

I like to use Arctic Char when wild salmon is unavailable. Arctic char is part of the salmon family, and according to the Environmental Defense Fund, it is less polluting to the environment than farmed salmon.

Steamed Arctic Char with Sautéed Leeks & Mushrooms

(pictured on page 95)

Serves 6

2 large leeks, white and light-green parts only, thinly sliced, then soaked in cold water to remove the grit

1 pound mushrooms, sliced

6 tablespoons salted butter

1/3 cup white wine plus more for the fish

Sea salt

Freshly ground black pepper

6 arctic char fillets (5 ounces each)

2 tablespoons chopped fresh flat-leaf parsley

2 tablespoons chopped fresh tarragon

1. Preheat the oven to 350°F.

2. Cut 6 pieces of parchment paper large enough to enclose each fillet.

3. Place some of the leeks and mushrooms on each piece of parchment. Add 1/2 tablespoon softened butter and 1 tablespoon of wine to each packet. Season with salt and pepper.

4. Place a piece of fish on top of the vegetables in each packet and season with salt and pepper. Rub 1/2 tablespoon softened butter onto each piece of fish.

5. Sprinkle the herbs over the fish and vegetables. Wrap each packet with the parchment paper so that fish and vegetables are fully enclosed.

6. Bake the packets for 15 to 25 minutes, or until the fish is cooked. Remove the baking sheet from the oven and let the fish rest for 5 minutes before serving on top of the leek and mushroom mixture.

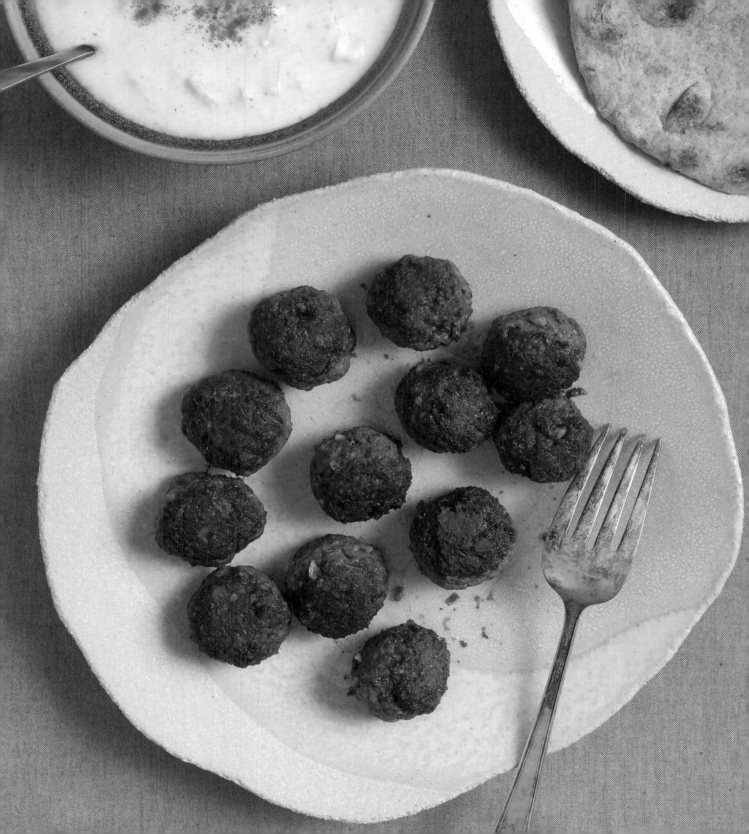

This is a delicious and innovative twist on the classic Italian meatball. The curry powder adds an unexpected layer of flavor, and the mango chutney offsets the spiciness nicely.

Indian-Spiced Meatballs

Serves 6 to 8

2 pounds ground lamb or beef

1 green serrano chile, seeded and chopped

6 garlic cloves, chopped

1 tablespoon grated fresh ginger

2 tablespoons curry powder

Sea salt

Freshly ground black pepper

1/4 cup grapeseed oil

6 to 8 whole-wheat pita or naan breads (optional)

Store-bought mango chutney, for serving

Cucumber raita, for serving (see recipe below)

1. If serving with pita or naan bread, preheat the oven to 250°F.

2. In a large bowl, combine the lamb or beef and the chile, garlic, ginger, curry powder, salt, and pepper and mix well.

3. Form the mixture into about 30 meatballs, each 1 inch in diameter.

4. Heat the oil in a large frying pan over medium-high heat. Add the meatballs in batches, and cook 8 to 12 minutes, until browned all over.

5. In the meantime, warm the pita or naan breads (if using) in the oven for 3 to 5 minutes.

6. Serve the meatballs with the bread, the mango chutney, and the cucumber raita.

Cucumber Raita

Makes 2 cups

2 cups plain full-fat yogurt (not Greek)

1 large cucumber, peeled, seeded, and diced

1/2 teaspoon roasted and ground cumin seeds

Sea salt

Freshly ground black pepper

Pinch of paprika, for garnish

Pinch of cayenne pepper, for garnish

1. In a medium bowl, whisk the yogurt until smooth.

2. Add the cucumber, cumin, salt, and pepper and mix well.

3. Transfer to a serving bowl and garnish with paprika and cayenne pepper.

This dish is quintessential comfort food, perfect on a cold winter evening. It takes some time to prepare, but the components can be made separately ahead of time, and it's a satisfying meal in and of itself.

Shepherd's Pie

Serves 6 to 8

4 tablespoons salted butter, plus more for the baking dish

2 pounds Yukon Gold potatoes, peeled and cut into large cubes

1 teaspoon sea salt, plus more for the pot

1/2 cup heavy cream

2 tablespoons extra-virgin olive oil

1 large onion, chopped

4 carrots, cut into 1/4-inch dice

2 garlic cloves, chopped

1 1/2 pounds ground lamb

1 cup chicken stock

1 cup crushed tomatoes, with their juice (from a glass jar*)

2 tablespoons Worcestershire sauce

1 teaspoon fresh thyme leaves

Freshly ground black pepper

1/2 to 1 cup grated Gruyère cheese

1. Preheat the oven to 400°F. Butter a 9x13-inch baking dish.

2. Put the potatoes in a large pot of cold, salted water. Bring to a boil, lower the heat to medium, and boil the potatoes until tender, 20 to 25 minutes; drain. Transfer to a medium heatproof bowl.

3. Meanwhile, heat the 4 tablespoons butter and the heavy cream in a small saucepan over low heat.

4. Add the melted butter and cream to the potatoes and mash with a potato masher until the butter and cream are well incorporated and the desired consistency is reached.

5. Heat the oil in a large sauté pan over medium heat. Add the onions, carrots, and garlic and sauté until soft, 10 to 12 minutes.

6. Add the lamb and cook, stirring, until browned. Stir in the stock, tomatoes, Worcestershire sauce, and thyme. Season with 1 teaspoon salt and pepper to taste. Simmer until the sauce has thickened slightly, about 25 minutes.

7. Transfer the lamb mixture to the prepared baking dish and spread in an even layer. Cover with the mashed potatoes, spreading in an even layer with a rubber spatula, then making peaks and swirls. Sprinkle the cheese over the top.

8. Bake for 30 minutes, until the potato topping starts to brown. Let sit for 10 minutes before serving.

*NOTE: I prefer to use crushed or diced tomatoes from glass jars rather than cans because the lining of many cans contains BPA, a chemical that has been linked to cancer, heart disease, and diabetes.

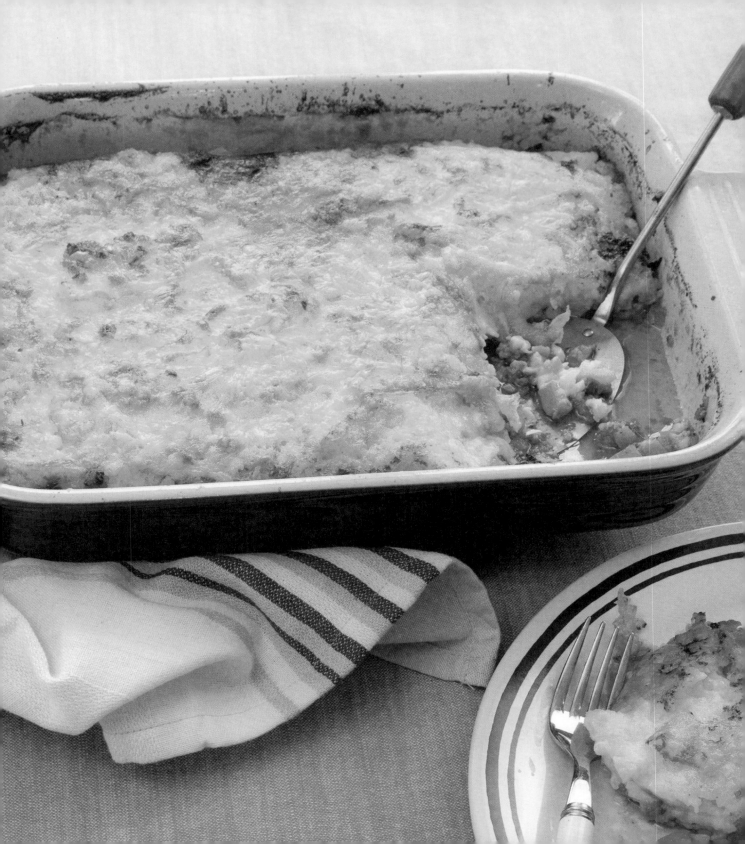

This versatile dish can be paired with a green salad and served as a simple midweek meal. Or it can be accompanied by one of the grain gratins on pages 107, 120, and 122, elevating it to weekend entertaining fare.

Sautéed Chicken Legs with Mustard Sauce

Serves 6

6 whole chicken legs

Sea salt

Freshly ground black pepper

2 to 4 tablespoons organic expeller-pressed sunflower oil

1 large onion, chopped

2 cups chicken or vegetable broth, white wine, or water

2 tablespoons Dijon mustard

2 teaspoons dry mustard

1/4 cup sliced fresh chives

1/4 cup crème fraîche

1. Season the chicken legs all over with salt and pepper.

2. Heat 2 tablespoons of the oil in a large sauté pan over medium-high heat. When hot, add the chicken and brown on both sides, 10 to 15 minutes total.

3. Remove the chicken from the pan and set aside. If the oil is too dark, wipe the pan with a paper towel and add 2 additional tablespoons of oil.

4. Add the onions to the pan and sauté until soft, about 5 minutes.

5. Add the broth, white wine, or water, Dijon mustard, and dry mustard. Mix well and bring to a boil.

6. Return the chicken to the pan. Cover, reduce heat to low, and simmer until the chicken legs are cooked through, 30 to 45 minutes. Remove the chicken to a serving platter and keep warm while you finish making the sauce.

7. Stir in the chives and crème fraîche and raise the heat to medium. Bring the sauce to a boil, then reduce the heat to low, and let simmer until it thickens, about 7 minutes. Pour the sauce over the chicken and serve immediately.

In India, this dish is typically made with ground lamb, but when my husband and daughter became vegetarians, I decided to try making it with tofu. It comes together very quickly and pairs beautifully with rice and dal, such as the "Khanna Dal" described on page 65.

Tofu Keema

Serves 6 to 8

3 tablespoons ghee or butter

1-inch stick of cinnamon

4 cardamom pods

2 bay leaves

1 medium onion, chopped

4 garlic cloves, chopped

1 tablespoon grated fresh ginger

1 1/2 to 2 pounds organic firm tofu, drained and patted dry

1 16-ounce package frozen peas, thawed

1/2 teaspoon turmeric

1 teaspoon garam masala

Pinch of cayenne pepper

2 tablespoons fresh lemon juice

Sea salt

Freshly ground black pepper

1. Heat the ghee in a large sauté pan over medium-high heat. When melted, stir in the cinnamon, cardamom, and bay leaves. Add the onions and fry until they are lightly browned, 5 to 7 minutes, then add the garlic and ginger. Sauté for a minute.

2. Add the tofu by crumbling it into the pan. The crumbles should be roughly the size of grains of rice. Sauté until lightly browned, about 5 more minutes.

3. Stir in the peas, turmeric, garam masala, cayenne pepper, lemon juice, salt, and black pepper.

4. Cook on low heat for an additional 10 minutes to allow the flavors to meld.

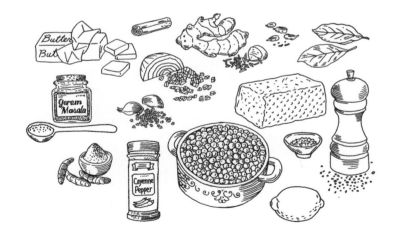

Because this sauce is so flavorful, I often serve it with something simple like mashed potatoes or rice pilaf. The sauce can be prepared 3 to 4 hours ahead of time and reheated when ready to spoon over the fish.

Roasted Halibut with Shallot & Saffron Sauce

Serves 6

1 cup thinly sliced shallots

1/4 cup extra-virgin olive oil

2 tablespoons balsamic vinegar

Sea salt

Freshly ground black pepper

2 pounds halibut fillets

1 tablespoon fresh thyme leaves

1 tablespoon finely grated lemon zest

1 cup clam juice

3/4 cup white wine

1/2 teaspoon crumbled saffron threads

Pinch of crushed red pepper flakes

2 tablespoons salted butter

1/4 cup crème fraîche (optional)

1. Preheat the oven to 325°F. Line a baking sheet with parchment paper. In a small bowl, combine the shallots, oil, and vinegar and mix well. Spread onto the prepared baking sheet. Season with salt and pepper.

2. Roast until the shallots are browned and soft, 15 to 20 minutes.

3. Remove the baking sheet from the oven and transfer the shallots to a small saucepan. Increase the oven temperature to 425°F. Line the baking sheet with a new piece of parchment paper. Arrange the fish on the baking sheet and season with salt and pepper, thyme, and lemon zest. Roast until the halibut is cooked through, 10 to 12 minutes.

4. In the meantime, into the saucepan with the shallots, add the clam juice, wine, saffron, and red pepper flakes. Bring to a boil, then reduce the heat to low, and simmer until the sauce thickens, 10 to 15 minutes. Stir in the butter and crème fraîche, if using.

5. Spoon the warm sauce over the fish before serving.

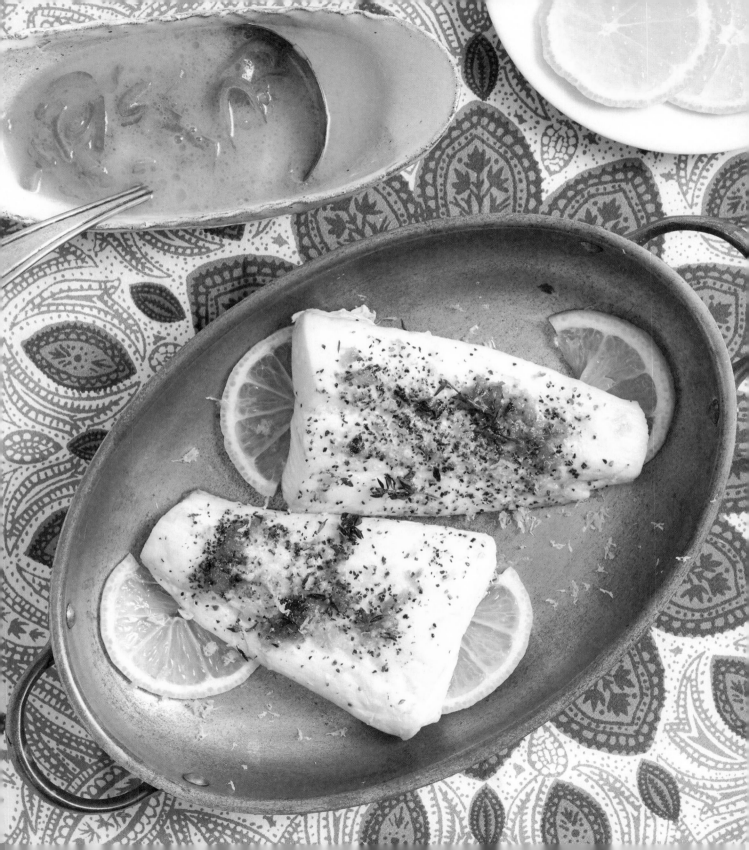

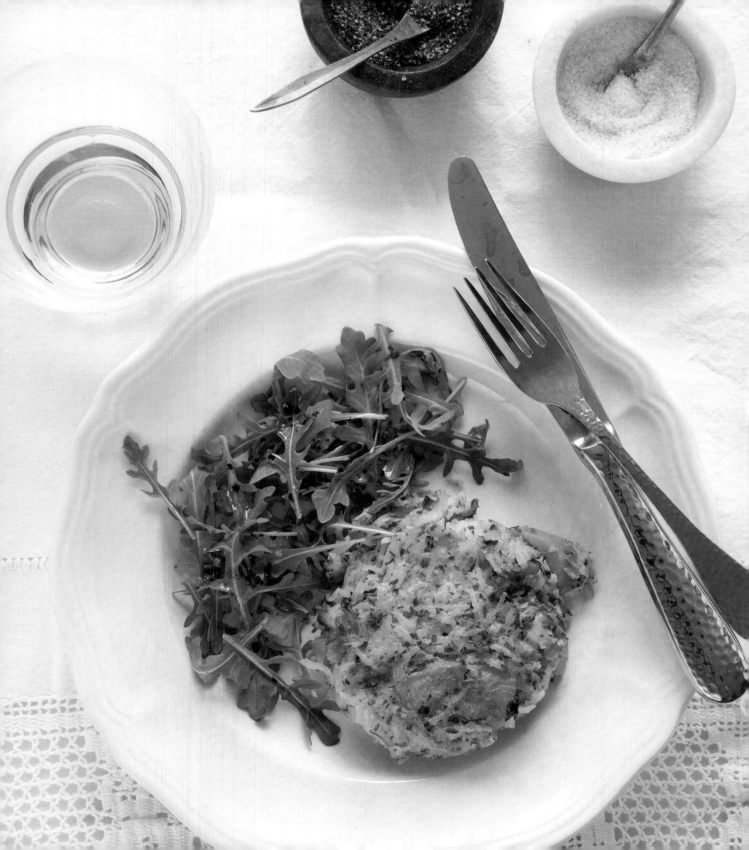

When I am looking for a dish that's warm and comforting on a cold day, this is the recipe I turn to. It takes a bit of time to make because you have to cook the rice, béchamel sauce, and vegetables separately but it is definitely worth the effort. And it is as good on the second day as it is on the first. It's filling enough that the only accompaniment you need is a simple green salad.

Rice Gratin with Carrots & Leeks

Serves 6 to 8

4 tablespoons salted butter, plus more for greasing the baking dish

I cup long-grain white or brown rice

2 cups whole, raw milk (pasteurized can be substituted)

1/2 small onion

I bay leaf

3 fresh thyme sprigs

1/4 cup all-purpose flour

Sea salt

Freshly ground black pepper

2 tablespoons olive oil

2 shallots, chopped

I pound leeks, white and light-green parts only, thinly sliced and then soaked in cold water to remove the grit

I pound carrots, thinly sliced on the diagonal

1/4 cup chopped fresh flat-leaf parsley

1/4 cup chopped fresh thyme

1/2 cup grated Parmigiano-Reggiano

1. Preheat the oven to 375°F. Butter a 9x13-inch baking dish.

2. Cook the rice according to the package directions. Set aside.

3. Make the béchamel sauce: Put the milk, onion, bay leaf, and thyme sprigs in a small pan and bring to a simmer over medium-low heat. Remove from the heat and let stand for 15 minutes, then strain, discarding the solids.

4. In a medium pot, melt the 4 tablespoons butter over low heat and add the flour. Whisk lightly, then add the strained milk. Cook over low heat, stirring constantly, until the mixture thickens and coats the back of a wooden spoon, 7 to 10 minutes. Season with salt and pepper and set aside.

5. Sauté the vegetables: In a medium sauté pan, heat the oil over medium heat. Add the shallots and cook until softened, about 3 minutes.

6. Add the leeks and carrots and sauté until lightly browned and soft, 10 to 12 minutes, stirring occasionally. You may need to lower the heat and cover the pan to allow the carrots to cook fully. Add the parsley and thyme and season with salt and pepper.

7. In a large bowl, combine the rice, béchamel sauce, vegetables, and cheese and mix well. Transfer to the prepared baking dish.

8. Bake until bubbling and browned, about 25 minutes.

Kicheree is a mixture of grains, usually rice and lentils, cooked together with spices to make porridge. I prefer when kicheree is very thick, but my husband likes it to be more like a soup, so this is clearly a matter of personal preference. It's often served when people have an upset stomach or are feeling unwell because it is very easy to digest and helps to support the immune system. I don't normally like to use pressure cookers, but I recommend using one for this recipe because a pressure cooker will make it easier to achieve the right consistency for the rice and mung beans without overcooking the vegetables. If you don't want to use a pressure cooker, I would recommend sautéing the vegetables separately and adding them at the end.

Kicheree

Serves 6 to 8

1 cup sprouted green mung beans

1 cup basmati rice

6 tablespoons ghee or butter

1/2 teaspoon black mustard seeds

1 teaspoon cumin seeds

1 teaspoon fennel seeds

8 curry leaves* (optional)

1 small onion, chopped

1 tablespoon grated garlic

1 tablespoon grated fresh ginger

1/4 cup 1/4-inch-diced carrots

1/4 cup cauliflower florets

1/4 cup 1/4-inch-diced potatoes

1/4 cup 1/4-inch-diced green beans

1 teaspoon turmeric

1 teaspoon sea salt

Freshly ground black pepper

1 teaspoon ground cumin

1 teaspoon ground coriander

1 teaspoon garam masala

1. Soak the mung beans and the rice in a bowl of water for 1 to 2 hours, changing the water at least once, to clean the beans and grains and remove some of the starch.

2. Heat 3 tablespoons of the ghee in a pressure cooker over medium heat. Add the black mustard, cumin, and fennel seeds, and the curry leaves, if using. When the spices start to pop, add the onion, garlic, and ginger. Sauté until lightly browned, 3 to 4 minutes.

3. Stir in the carrots, cauliflower, potatoes, green beans, and turmeric and season with salt and pepper. Sauté for 2 to 3 minutes.

4. Drain the rice and mung beans and add to the pressure cooker with 8 cups of water. Lock the cover on the pressure cooker and set the pressure to high. Cook on high pressure for 5 minutes, then release the pressure manually.

5. The kicheree will have a thick consistency, but if you prefer it soupier, add more water to thin it out. Mix in the sautéed vegetables.

6. While the kicheree is cooking, heat the remaining 3 tablespoons of ghee in a small sauté pan. Add the ground cumin and coriander, and the garam masala and stir for 30 seconds. Drizzle on top of the kicheree before serving.

*NOTE: Curry leaves can be found in most specialty Indian food stores or online.

After a long hard winter, there are many reasons to welcome spring. Not least of which is that spring brings with it asparagus and ramp season. Ramps have an especially short season so I love to put them to as many uses as possible as soon as I see them.

Asparagus Risotto with Ramp Pesto

Serves 6

FOR THE PESTO

1 teaspoon sea salt, plus more for the water

8 ounces ramps*

1/2 cup whole walnuts, lightly toasted

2/3 cup extra-virgin olive oil

1/4 cup grated Parmiggiano-Reggiano

Sea salt

FOR THE RISOTTO

6 cups warm vegetable broth

2 tablespoons salted butter

1 medium onion, chopped

2 cups arborio or vialone nano rice

1/2 cup white wine

1 cup ramp cooking water, reserved from the pesto

2 bunches asparagus, trimmed and cut into 1/2-inch pieces

1 cup grated Parmiggiano-Reggiano

1/4 cup heavy cream

Sea salt

Freshly ground black pepper

*A NOTE ON RAMPS: If ramps are not in season, substitute the same quantity of scallions, garlic, garlic scapes, or some combination of the three. If substituting ramps, omit step 1.

MAKE THE PESTO

1. Bring a large pot of salted water to a boil. Cut the greens from the ramps and reserve the bulbs. Blanch the greens in a large pot until just wilted. Drain, reserving 1 cup of the cooking water for the risotto.

2. Coarsely chop the bulbs. Combine the ramp greens, ramp bulbs, walnuts, oil, cheese, and 1 teaspoon salt in a blender and process to a smooth paste.

MAKE THE RISOTTO

1. Pour the broth into a medium saucepan and bring to a simmer over medium-low heat.

2. Melt the butter in a large saucepan over medium heat. Add the onions and sauté until soft and translucent, 3 to 5 minutes.

3. Add the rice and stir until well coated with the butter. Add the wine and simmer until fully absorbed, about 4 minutes.

4. Add the warm broth and reserved ramp cooking water to the rice, a ladleful at a time, stirring continuously. Allow the liquid to be fully absorbed before adding the next ladleful; it should take about 2 minutes to absorb each ladleful. Cook, continuing to stir and add broth, for 12 to 15 minutes.

5. Add the asparagus pieces and continue adding the broth until the rice is tender but still has a hint of crunch, an additional 8 to 10 minutes. Stir in the ramp pesto.

6. Add the cheese and cream and mix well. Season with salt and pepper to taste and serve immediately.

Risotto, much like Indian kicheree or Chinese congee, is full of vitamins and easy on the digestive system. And it doesn't hurt that it tastes great, too.

Artichoke Risotto

Serves 6 to 8

6 cups chicken or vegetable broth

4 tablespoons salted butter

1 medium onion, finely chopped

2 cups arborio or vialone nano rice

1/2 cup white wine

8-ounce jar of roasted artichoke hearts, drained

1/2 cup grated Parmigiano-Reggiano

Sea salt

Freshly ground black pepper

2 tablespoons chopped fresh flat-leaf parsley

1. Pour the broth into a medium saucepan and bring to a simmer over medium-low heat.

2. Melt 2 tablespoons of the butter in a large saucepan over medium heat. Add the onion and cook until translucent, about 5 minutes.

3. Add the rice and stir until well coated with the butter. Add the wine and simmer until fully absorbed, about 4 minutes.

4. Add the warm broth to the rice, a ladleful at a time, stirring continuously. Allow the liquid to be fully absorbed before adding the next ladleful; it should take about 2 minutes.

5. Add the artichoke and continue adding the broth until the rice is tender but still has a hint of crunch, an additional 8 to 10 minutes.

6. When the rice is done, add the remaining 2 tablespoons butter and the cheese and quickly stir them in. Garnish with parsley, adjust seasoning, and serve immediately.

NOTE: Either of these risottos can be made with farro or barley, if you prefer.

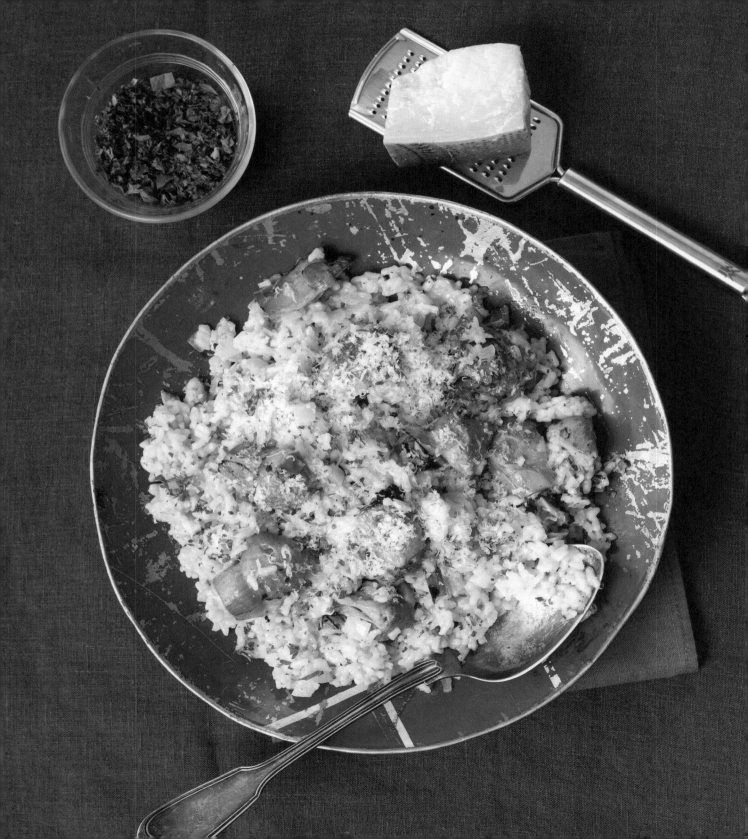

The Formula: **Grain Bowls**

Grain bowls, accompanied by a simple side salad, are a great lunch or dinner option as they contain all the macronutrients one needs. Because grain bowls can be enjoyed hot or at room temperature, you can prepare the ingredients ahead of time at your leisure and then combine them when you are ready to eat. **Serves 4**

1. Choose the grain

(1 cup of uncooked grain)

Select a grain that will hold up and not get mushy, such as:

brown rice

farro

barley

quinoa

Cook the selected grain according to package directions.

2. Choose the vegetable

(1 pound)

steamed cauliflower

roasted sweet potatoes, beets, squash, and other root vegetables

sautéed spinach and mushrooms

3. Choose the spice(s)

Some versatile ones include:

1 teaspoon curry powder

1/2 teaspoon paprika

1 teaspoon ground cumin

pinch of cayenne

Mix the vegetables with the chosen spices.

4. Choose the protein (optional)

If you'd like, choose a protein to add to the grain bowl. Some good choices are:

hard-boiled eggs

steamed or poached chicken breast

roasted fish

5. Make a light vinaigrette

See page 113 for some suggestions.

6. Assemble the grain bowl

Put 1/2 cup of the cooked grain into each of the four bowls. Top with the spiced vegetable(s) and protein, if using.

Dress the grain bowl about 20 to 30 minutes before serving so the flavors have time to meld.

Recommended combinations include:

- Brown rice with steamed cauliflower and curry vinaigrette

- Farro with paprika-spiced roasted root vegetables and balsamic vinaigrette

- Barley with sautéed spinach and mushrooms and herb & shallot vinaigrette

- Quinoa with roasted sweet potatoes and lime-cilantro vinaigrette

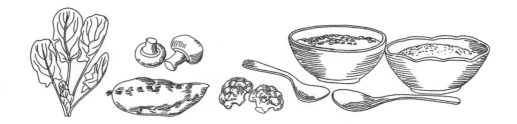

Curry Vinaigrette

Makes 1/2 to 3/4 cup

2 tablespoons apple cider vinegar

1 tablespoon curry powder

1 garlic clove, grated

1/2 cup extra-virgin olive oil

Salt

Freshly ground black pepper

1. In a small bowl, combine the vinegar, curry powder, and garlic and mix well.
2. Add the oil and whisk until fully combined. Season with salt and pepper.

Herb & Shallot Vinaigrette

Makes about 1/2 cup

2 tablespoons white wine vinegar

1 large shallot, finely chopped

1/4 cup chopped herbs, such as parsley, chives, and tarragon

6 tablespoons extra-virgin olive oil

Salt

Freshly ground black pepper

1. In a small bowl, combine the vinegar and shallot and mix well.
2. Add the oil and whisk until fully combined. Season with salt and pepper.

Lime-Cilantro Vinaigrette

Makes 1/2 to 3/4 cup

2 tablespoons fresh lime juice

1/2 cup extra-virgin olive oil

1 teaspoon finely grated lime zest

1/4 teaspoon cayenne pepper (optional)

1/4 cup chopped fresh cilantro

Salt

Freshly ground black pepper

1. In a small bowl, whisk the lime juice and oil until well combined.
2. Add the zest, cayenne pepper, and cilantro and whisk again. Season with salt and pepper.

Balsamic Vinaigrette

Makes 1/2 to 3/4 cup

2 tablespoons balsamic vinegar

1/2 teaspoon Dijon mustard

1/2 cup extra-virgin olive oil

Salt

Freshly ground black pepper

1. In a small bowl, combine the vinegar and mustard and mix well.
2. Add the oil and whisk until fully combined. Season with salt and pepper.

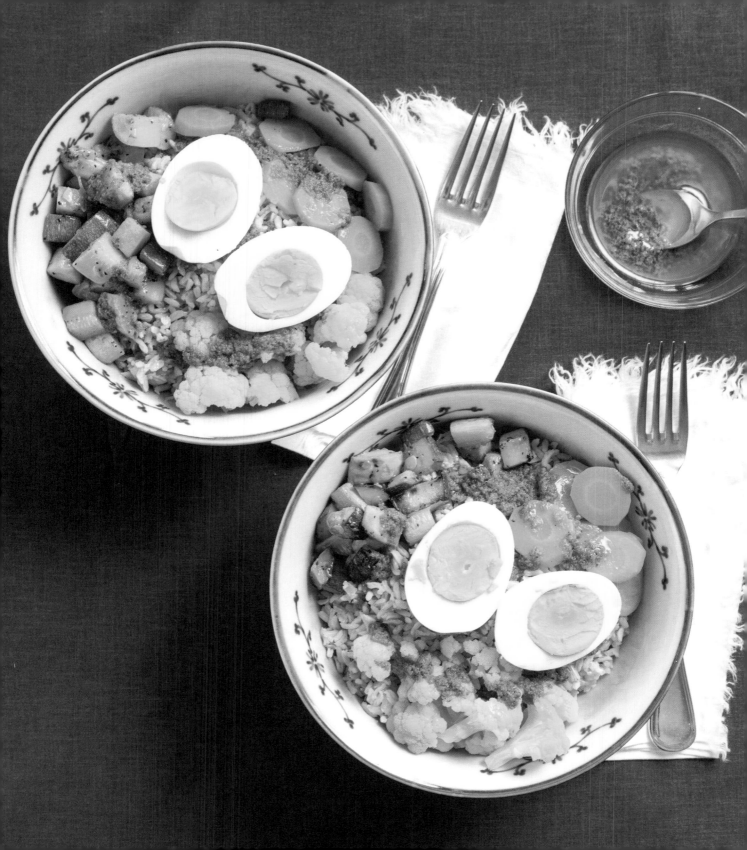

My favorite thing about grain bowls is that they're a creative way to use up any leftovers in your refrigerator. Just add an interesting dressing to some leftover quinoa or rice or sautéed vegetables, and you have a whole new dish!

Brown Rice Bowl with Zucchini, Carrots, Cauliflower & Hard-Boiled Eggs

Serves 2

1 tablespoon olive oil

2 small zucchini, quartered lengthwise, then cut crosswise into 1/2-inch pieces

Sea salt

2 carrots, peeled and sliced into thin rounds

1/2 small head of cauliflower, cut into bite-size florets

1 cup cooked brown rice

2 hard-boiled eggs, halved lengthwise

Curry Vinaigrette (see page 113)

1. Heat the oil in a small sauté pan over medium heat. Add the zucchini and sauté until soft and lightly browned. Set aside.

2. Bring a medium pot of salted water to a boil over medium heat. Boil the carrots until soft, 5 to 7 minutes. Remove the carrots with a slotted spoon and set aside.

3. Return the water in the pot to a boil and add the cauliflower. Boil the cauliflower until soft, 7 to 9 minutes. Remove with a slotted spoon and set aside.

4. Divide the rice into two small bowls. Top each bowl with half the zucchini, carrots, and cauliflower, then the hard-boiled egg halves.

5. Drizzle on some dressing and let sit for 20 to 30 minutes so the flavors meld. Serve warm or at room temperature.

I recently started experimenting with the ancient cracked grain freekeh. It is similar to bulgur, but to me it has a richer flavor. Researchers in Australia found that, because freekeh is harvested when it's young, the grain retains more protein, fiber, and minerals than regular wheat. Freekeh is also said to have more fiber than brown rice or quinoa. These "meatballs" are inspired by a recipe on www.freekehlicious.com. You can serve them with spaghetti and homemade or store-bought marinara sauce or simply enjoy them accompanied by a green salad.

Freekeh "Meatballs"

Serves 6

1 cup cracked freekeh*

3 1/2 cups vegetable broth

2 tablespoons extra-virgin olive oil

1 medium onion, finely chopped

2 garlic cloves, finely chopped

3/4 cup sourdough breadcrumbs**

1/2 cup grated Parmigiano-Reggiano

1/2 cup grated Pecorino-Romano

3 large eggs, lightly whisked

1 tablespoon fresh thyme leaves

Sea salt

Freshly ground black pepper

1. Combine the freekeh and broth in a medium pot. Bring to a boil, stir, and reduce the heat to low. Cover the pot and cook for 20 minutes. Remove from the heat and let cool. (This step is best done about 1 hour ahead of time so that the freekeh can cool completely.)

2. Preheat the oven to 400°F. Line a rimmed baking sheet with parchment paper and brush it with oil.

3. Once cool, in a large bowl, combine the freekeh, onions, garlic, breadcrumbs, cheeses, eggs, thyme, salt, and pepper and mix well.

4. Form the freekeh mixture into golf-ball-size "meatballs" and place them on the baking sheet. Bake for 20 minutes, then turn the "meatballs" over, and bake for an additional 5 to 10 minutes. They should be nicely browned on all sides.

*NOTE: Freekeh can be found in most specialty food stores or online.

**A NOTE ON BREADCRUMBS: You can make your own breadcrumbs by taking some stale bread and rubbing it with your fingers until it makes crumbs. For finer breadcrumbs, use a mortar and pestle or food processor. Place crumbs on a baking sheet and toast in a 350°F oven for 10 to 15 minutes, until the crumbs turn golden.

It's always helpful when I can find new ways to incorporate different grains into our diet, especially since I am not a big fan of rice. Given that quinoa can be a little flavorless on its own, I like it in this adaptation of fried rice.

Quinoa Fried Rice

Serves 6 to 8

1 1/2 cups quinoa, soaked overnight

2 tablespoons plus 2 teaspoons extra-virgin olive oil

2 large eggs, beaten

8 ounces shiitake mushrooms, thinly sliced

1 cup 1/4-inch-diced carrot

1 cup 1/4-inch-diced celery

1 red bell pepper, seeded and cut into 1/4-inch dice

1 cup broccoli, cut into small florets

4 garlic cloves, chopped

1/4 cup grated fresh ginger

1 1/2 cups frozen shelled edamame, thawed

3 tablespoons tamari

2 scallions (white and green parts), thinly sliced

1. Cook the quinoa according to package directions. Set aside and let cool.

2. Heat a wok or large sauté pan over medium heat. Add 1 teaspoon of the oil, then add half the eggs. Swirl the pan so that there is a thin layer of egg along the bottom. Cook for 30 seconds, flip the egg over, cook for another 15 seconds, then transfer to a small cutting board. Repeat with 1 teaspoon oil and the remaining egg. Put one egg "pancake" on top of the other, roll them up, and slice into thin strips.

3. Wipe the pan clean and add the remaining 2 tablespoons oil. Add the mushrooms, carrots, celery, red pepper, and broccoli. Cook over medium heat until the vegetables soften, 5 to 6 minutes. Stir in the garlic and ginger and cook 1 minute more.

4. Add the quinoa and mix well. Continue cooking over medium heat until the quinoa is fully reheated, about 5 minutes. Add the egg, edamame, and tamari sauce and mix well.

5. Garnish with the scallions and serve.

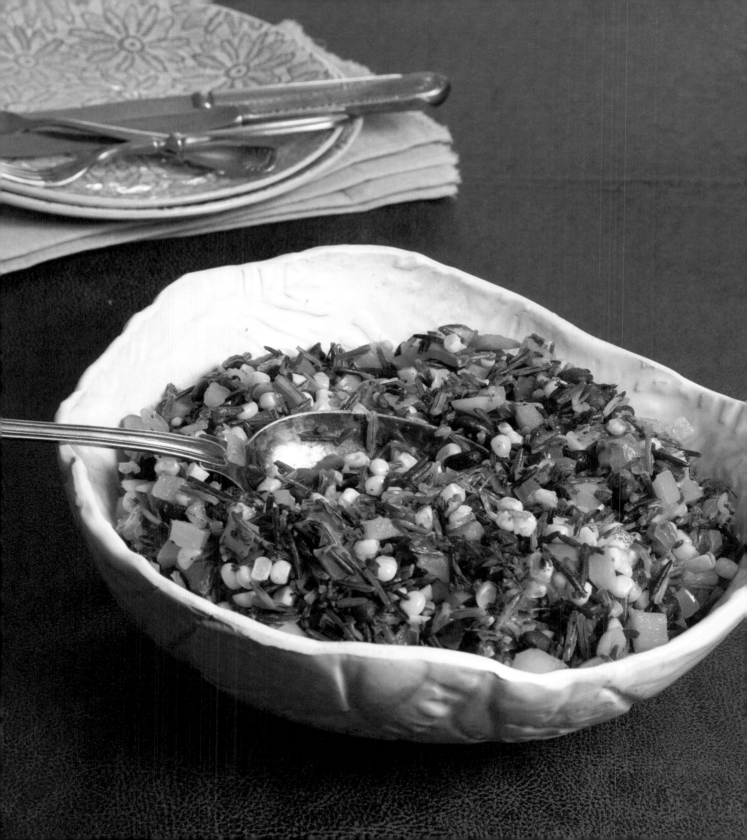

I came up with this variation of rice and beans for my vegetarian husband and daughter. I like how the nuttiness of the wild rice combines with the sweetness of the sautéed vegetables.

Wild Rice with Black Beans, Peppers & Corn

Serves 6

1/4 cup extra-virgin olive oil

1 large red onion, chopped

2 red bell peppers, seeded and cut into 1/4-inch dice

1 ear of corn, kernels removed

1 cup wild rice, cooked according to package directions*

1 1/2 cups (or 2 cans) cooked black beans

3 dashes Tabasco sauce (optional)

Sea salt

Freshly ground black pepper

1/4 cup chopped fresh cilantro

1. Heat the oil in a large sauté pan over medium heat. Sauté the onion until soft, 3 to 5 minutes.

2. Add the red peppers and corn and continue sautéing until soft, another 3 to 5 minutes.

3. Add the rice and beans and cook, stirring often, until they are heated through.

4. Season with Tabasco, if using, and salt and pepper.

5. Sprinkle with the cilantro and serve.

*NOTE: There are many delicious varieties of heritage wild rice. I would recommend using one of these to support growers of heritage breeds.

Since my husband became a vegetarian, I've been experimenting with different dishes to make sure that he gets enough protein. This dish certainly fits the bill. It's filling and delicious, and loaded with protein.

Farro, Spinach & Cheese Gratin

Serves 6

Salted butter, for greasing the baking dish

1 cup heavy cream

1 cup mascarpone cheese

4 ounces Gorgonzola (preferably creamy), cut into small pieces

Sea salt

Freshly ground black pepper

2 pounds spinach, thick stems trimmed

2 tablespoons extra-virgin olive oil

1/2 cup thinly sliced scallions

2 garlic cloves, chopped

2 tablespoons chopped fresh dill

2 tablespoons chopped fresh flat-leaf parsley

1 cup farro, cooked according to package directions

1. Preheat the oven to 400°F. Butter a 9x13-inch baking dish.

2. In a small saucepan, combine the cream, mascarpone, and Gorgonzola. Cook over low heat until the cheeses melt, about 5 minutes. Season with salt and pepper and set aside.

3. Bring a medium pot of salted water to a boil. Add the spinach and boil until wilted, 3 to 4 minutes. Drain, rinse under cold water, squeeze out the excess water, and chop.

4. Heat the oil in a large sauté pan. When hot, add the spinach, scallions, garlic, dill, and parsley. Sauté until the spinach is wilted, 3 to 4 minutes. Season with salt and pepper.

5. In a large bowl, combine the spinach mixture, farro, and cheese mixture. Mix well and pour into the prepared baking dish.

6. Bake until lightly browned, about 25 minutes.

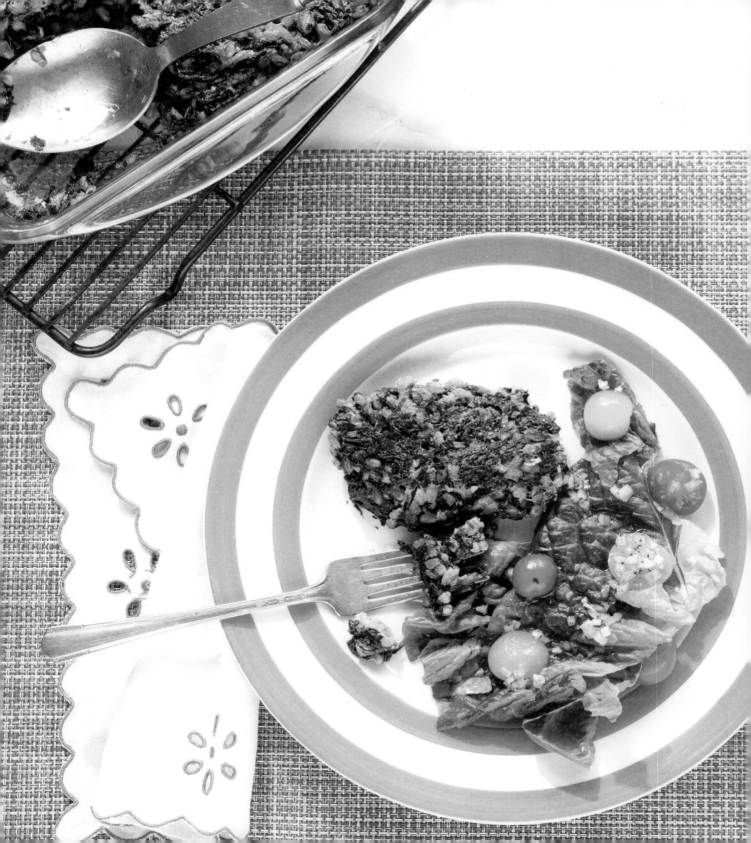

This recipe is adapted from one in Deborah Madison's Vegetarian Cooking for Everyone. When my husband first became a vegetarian, I found I was cooking a lot of rice. In my search for alternative grain options, I found that farro gave this recipe a nice earthy flavor that I even preferred to rice.

Zucchini & Farro Gratin

Serves 6 to 8

4 tablespoons salted butter, plus more for the baking dish

2 cups raw whole milk (pasteurized can be substituted)

2 medium onions, 1 quartered and 1 chopped

1 bay leaf

3 sprigs fresh flat-leaf parsley plus 1/4 cup chopped

2 sprigs fresh thyme plus 1/4 cup leaves

1/4 cup all-purpose flour

1/4 cup chopped fresh tarragon

Sea salt

Freshly ground black pepper

1 1/2 pounds zucchini and/or yellow squash, grated

2 tablespoons extra-virgin olive oil

1 cup farro, cooked according to package directions

1/2 cup grated Parmigiano-Reggiano

1. Preheat the oven to 375°F. Butter a 9x13-inch baking dish.

2. Make the béchamel: Put the milk, the quartered onion, the bay leaf, and the parsley and thyme sprigs in a small pan and bring to a simmer over medium-low heat. Remove from the heat and let stand for 15 minutes, then strain; discard the solids.

3. In another pan, combine the 4 tablespoons butter and the flour and cook over low heat, until butter melts. Stir until the mixture resembles coarse sand then add the strained milk. Cook over low heat, stirring constantly, until the mixture thickens and coats the back of a wooden spoon, about 10 minutes. Add the chopped tarragon and parsley and the thyme leaves to the béchamel, season with salt and pepper, and set aside.

4. Combine the zucchini with 1 teaspoon salt and set aside in a colander to remove excess water.

5. Heat the oil in a large sauté pan over medium heat. Sauté the chopped onions until soft but not browned, about 5 minutes. Add the zucchini and continue to sauté, stirring occasionally, until lightly browned, about 10 minutes. Season with salt and pepper.

6. In a large bowl, combine the zucchini with the farro and béchamel and mix well. Transfer to the baking dish and sprinkle the cheese on top.

7. Bake until the top is nicely browned, about 25 minutes.

A mujadara is a spiced rice and lentil dish from the Middle East. This is adapted from the classic recipe. Here, I use butternut squash and turnips, but you could use any mix of root vegetables, such as beets, carrots, or pumpkin. Accompanied by a salad, this makes a satisfying midweek vegetarian meal.

Mujadara with Butternut Squash & Turnips

Serves 6 to 8

I cup brown lentils

1/4 cup extra-virgin olive oil

2 leeks, white and light-green parts only, thinly sliced, then soaked in cold water to remove the grit

2 garlic cloves, chopped

3/4 cup basmati rice

I 1/2 teaspoons ground cumin

1/2 teaspoon ground allspice

Pinch of cayenne pepper

I cup 1/2-inch-cubed butternut squash

I cup 1/2-inch-cubed turnips

2 teaspoons sea salt

I bay leaf

I cinnamon stick

4 cups kale, stems removed and leaves thinly sliced

1. Put the lentils in a small bowl and cover with warm water. Let them soak while you prepare the remaining ingredients.

2. Heat the oil in a large pot over medium heat. Add the leeks and cook until browned, stirring occasionally, 5 to 7 minutes.

3. Add the garlic and rice and stir until coated with oil. Stir in the cumin, allspice, and cayenne.

4. Drain the lentils and add them to the pot, along with the squash and turnips. Add 4 cups water, the salt, bay leaf, and cinnamon. Bring to a boil. Cover, reduce the heat to low, and cook for 15 minutes.

5. Add the kale, mix well, and simmer until the rice is cooked and the kale is wilted, an additional 5 to 7 minutes.

I love any yogurt and cucumber combination, especially in summer, because it is so cooling. This tzatziki adds a bright note to the earthy mujardara above.

Tzatziki

Makes 2 cups

16 ounces Greek yogurt

2 English cucumbers, peeled, seeded, and grated

I tablespoon chopped fresh dill

2 garlic cloves, grated

2 tablespoons extra-virgin olive oil

Sea salt

Freshly ground black pepper

1. In a small bowl, combine the yogurt, cucumbers, dill, garlic, and oil and mix well. Season with salt and pepper.

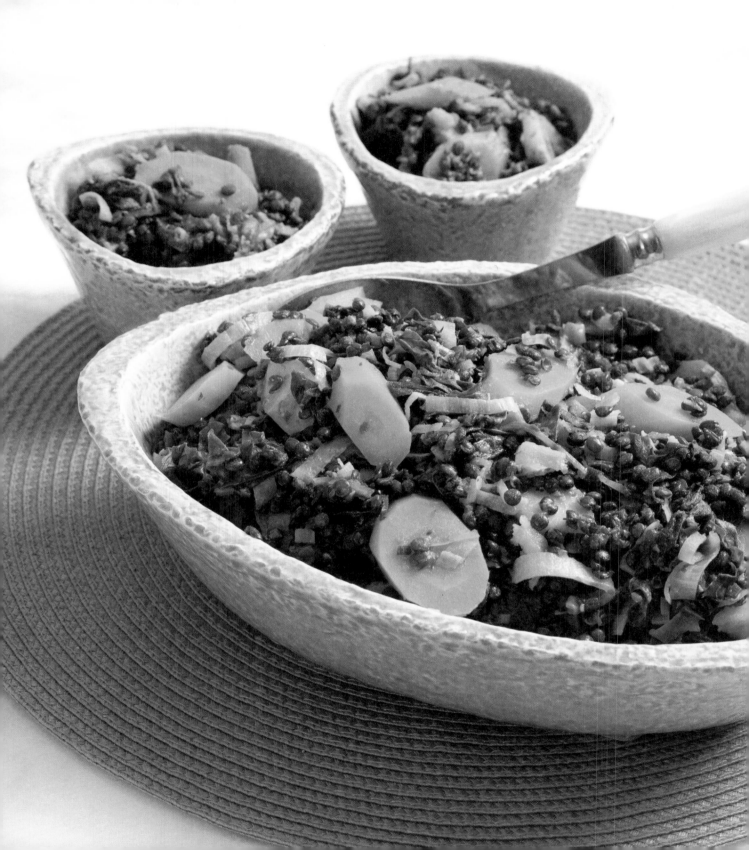

While I generally associate lentils with winter, I think this is a delicious dish for any time of year. You can make it more seasonal by changing the mix of vegetables, using root vegetables in winter; spring onions, sugar snap or snow peas, and asparagus in spring; zucchini, summer squash, and green beans in summer.

Beluga Lentils with Leeks, Carrots, Parsnips & Chard

Serves 6 to 8

1 1/2 cups beluga (black) lentils

Sea salt

5 tablespoons salted butter, at room temperature

2 leeks, white and light-green parts only, thinly sliced, then soaked in cold water to remove the grit

3 carrots, thinly sliced

3 parsnips, peeled and thinly sliced

1 teaspoon grainy mustard

1 teaspoon fresh lemon juice

3/4 cup vegetable broth

1 bunch Swiss chard, stems removed and leaves sliced into thin strips

1 tablespoon sliced fresh chives

1 teaspoon chopped fresh tarragon

Freshly ground black pepper

1. Combine the lentils, 6 cups water, and salt in a large pot. Bring to a boil, reduce the heat to low, and simmer until the lentils are cooked, about 25 minutes. Drain and set aside.

2. Rinse the pot, return it to medium-low heat, and melt 2 tablespoons of the butter. Add the leeks, carrots, and parsnips and sauté for 3 to 4 minutes. Cover, reduce the heat to low, and cook an additional 5 minutes, stirring occasionally, until the carrots and parsnips are soft.

3. In a small bowl, mix the remaining 3 tablespoons butter with the mustard and lemon juice.

4. Add the lentils, mustard-butter mixture, broth, Swiss chard, chives, and tarragon to the vegetable pot and cook over low heat, stirring occasionally, until the chard is wilted, an additional 5 to 6 minutes. Season with salt and pepper.

I had a version of this dish during a trip to Switzerland. I loved it so much, I decided to develop my own version. It's satisfying without being too heavy to digest.

Sautéed Lima Beans, Kale, Carrots & Turnips

Serves 6

1 cup dried baby green lima beans, soaked overnight, then drained

Sea salt

4 tablespoons salted butter

4 carrots, cut into small dice

2 turnips, cut into small dice

1/2 to 1 cup vegetable broth

1 bunch kale, stems removed and leaves coarsely chopped

Freshly ground black pepper

1/4 cup chopped fresh flat-leaf parsley

1. Put the lima beans in a medium pot of salted water. Bring to a boil, reduce the heat, and cook until soft but not mushy, 30 to 45 minutes. Drain and set aside.

2. Melt the butter in a large sauté pan over medium-low heat. Add the carrots and turnips and sauté until soft and well coated with butter, 2 to 3 minutes. Add enough broth to come halfway up the side of the pan.

3. Cover, reduce the heat to low, and cook until the broth has almost evaporated, about 7 minutes.

4. Add the kale and continue to cook over low heat, stirring occasionally, until it is wilted, 5 to 7 minutes.

5. Stir in the beans and continue cooking over low heat until reheated. Season with salt and pepper. Stir in the parsley and serve.

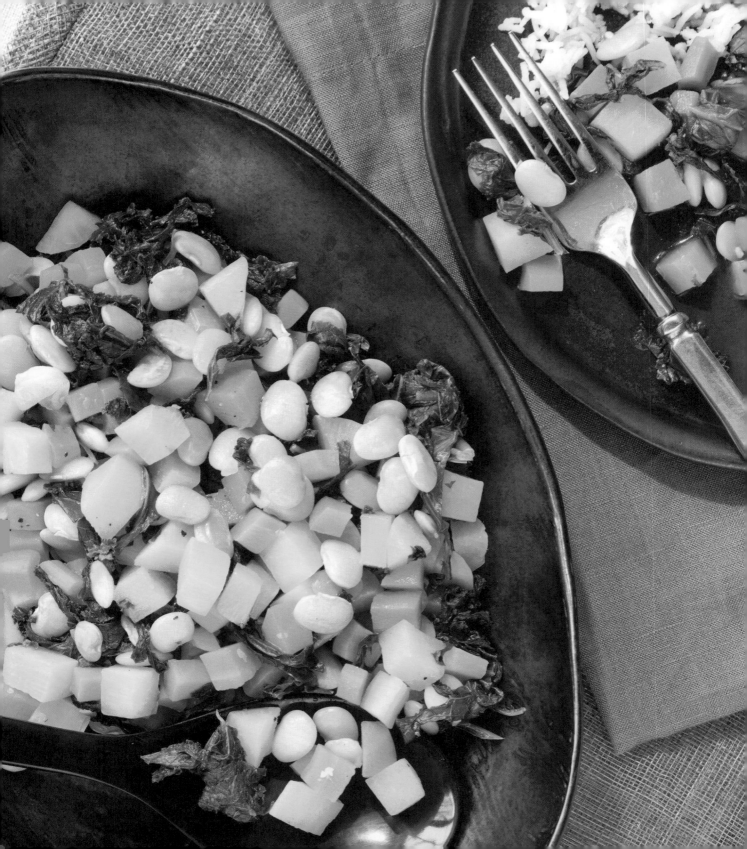

Falafel are typically served with tahini sauce; however, I prefer to serve them with tzatziki on the side (see recipe on page 123). I add squash to my falafel mixture to make them a meal on their own, but they also go beautifully with a side of roasted root vegetables.

Oven-Baked Squash Falafel

Serves 6 to 8

2 cups dried chickpeas, soaked overnight

1 1/2 to 2 cups butternut squash or pumpkin purée*

2 garlic cloves, chopped

1 medium onion, quartered

1/2 cup fresh cilantro

1/2 cup fresh flat-leaf parsley

1 teaspoon sea salt

1 teaspoon ground cumin

1/2 teaspoon ground coriander

Pinch of paprika

1/2 teaspoon baking soda

1/2 teaspoon freshly ground black pepper

1/4 cup extra-virgin olive oil

1. In a food processor, purée the chickpeas with the squash, garlic, onion, cilantro, parsley, salt, cumin, coriander, paprika, baking soda, and pepper until smooth. Spread the purée onto a large rimmed baking sheet and refrigerate, uncovered, for about 1 hour so that the mixture hardens and is easier to roll.

2. Preheat the oven to 375°F.

3. Grease another baking sheet with 2 tablespoons of the oil. Roll the chickpea mixture into twenty 1 1/2-inch balls. Lay the balls on the baking sheet and flatten them slightly. Make a small thumb imprint in the middle of each patty.

4. Drizzle the remaining 2 tablespoons oil on top of the patties

5. Bake until lightly browned, 10 to 15 minutes. Serve with tahini or the tzatziki on page 121.

*NOTE: To make puréed squash or pumpkin, preheat the oven to 350°F. Cut a butternut squash or pumpkin in half, remove the seeds, pour a little olive oil on the cut side. Roast cut side down, until soft, 1 to 1 1/2 hours. Scrape out the inside and purée with a potato masher or in a blender until smooth.

This is my take on a recipe in Deborah Madison's Vegetarian Cooking for Everyone. *I would serve this with either of the kale salads on pages 80 and 81 or simply with some sautéed greens with garlic and red pepper flakes.*

Winter Vegetable Pot Pie

Serves 6 to 8

4 tablespoons salted butter

2 tablespoons extra-virgin olive oil

1 1/2 pounds butternut squash, peeled and cut into 1-inch cubes

6 small shallots, halved

1 celery root, peeled and cut into 3/4-inch cubes

2 beets, peeled and cut into 3/4-inch cubes

6 carrots, sliced into 1-inch pieces on the diagonal

Sea salt

Freshly ground black pepper

2 cups heavy cream

1/4 cup chopped fresh flat-leaf parsley

1/4 cup chopped fresh tarragon

1/4 cup thyme leaves

1 sheet (about 14 ounces) frozen puff pastry, thawed

All-purpose flour for rolling the pastry

1 large egg, beaten

1. Heat 3 tablespoons of the butter and the oil in a large sauté pan over medium heat. Add the squash, shallots, celery root, beets, and carrots. Sauté until lightly browned, about 5 minutes.

2. Cover, reduce the heat to low, and cook, stirring occasionally, until the vegetables are soft but have a hint of firmness left, 15 to 20 minutes. If the vegetables begin to stick to the pan, add a little water. Season with salt and pepper. Remove from the heat and set aside.

3. Meanwhile, heat the cream in a small saucepan over medium-high heat. Bring to a boil and let cook until the cream has reduced and thickened slightly, 5 to 7 minutes. Remove from the heat and add the herbs.

4. Preheat the oven to 425°F. Butter a baking dish or pie plate* large enough to hold all the vegetables. Place the vegetables in the baking dish. Add the cream and combine. Roll out the puff pastry on a floured board until it is about 1/4 inch thick. Cut it to fit over the top of the dish, overlapping a little. Using a pairing knife, make small cuts in the pastry to let the steam escape. If there is extra, cut out small shapes to decorate the top of the pastry.

5. Cover the vegetables with the puff pastry and brush the top with the egg. Press any dough cutouts on top and brush with more egg.

6. Bake for 12 minutes. Reduce the heat to 350°F and bake until the pastry is browned and the filling is bubbling, an additional 10 to 15 minutes.

7. Remove from the oven and let cool for 5 to 10 minutes before serving.

*NOTE: For an alternative presentation, you can serve this in individual gratin dishes.

Sides

These fresh, flavorful side dishes can accompany any of the entrées. Alternatively, they can be paired with a steamed whole grain and a salad to become a meal.

Sauteed Onions, Carrots, Fennel & Cabbage with Preserved Lemons, recipe on page 144 ››

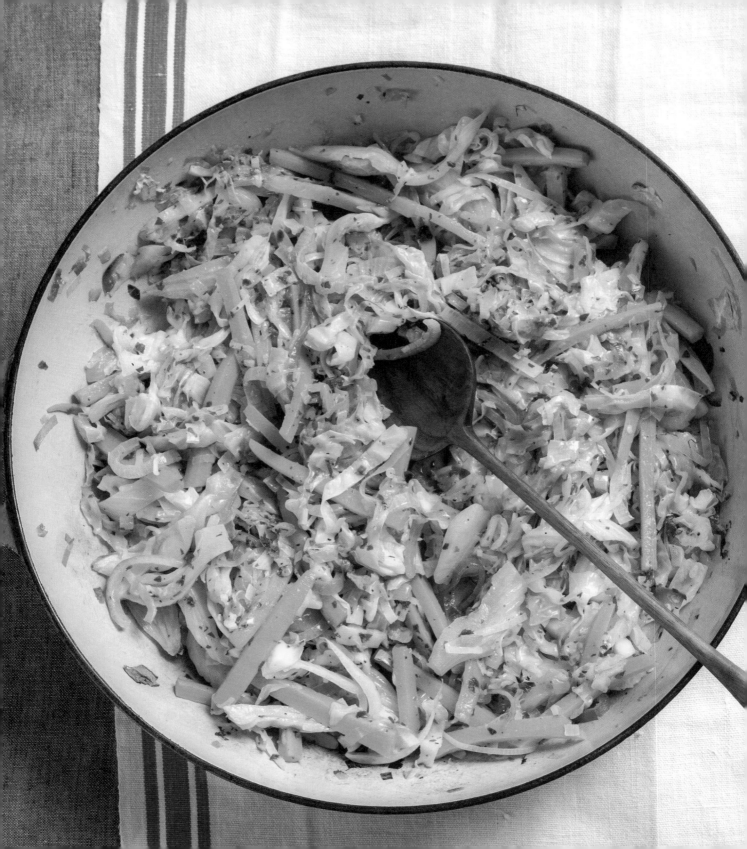

The Formula: Sautéed Vegetables

Sautéed vegetables are my go-to side dish when I want to whip up something quickly using the seasonal vegetables I invariably have in the fridge. **Serves 6**

1. Choose the allium
(1 cup chopped)

red or yellow onion

shallots

2. Choose the vegetable combination (about 2 cups)

carrots and parsnips

carrots, asparagus, and snap peas

zucchini, yellow squash, red pepper, and corn

3. Choose the herbs
(2 tablespoons)

parsley

tarragon

chives

cilantro

4. Plus basic ingredients

4 tablespoons olive oil

sea salt and freshly ground black pepper

5. Make the sautéed vegetables

1. Heat the oil over medium heat in a medium sauté pan. Add the allium and sauté until soft, 3 to 5 minutes.

2. Add the vegetables that will take the most time to cook and sauté 3 to 5 minutes. Reduce the heat to low, cover the pan and cook another 3 minutes.

3. Add the vegetables that will cook faster; continue to sauté until all the vegetables are soft.

4. Stir in herbs and/or seasonings.

5. Season with sea salt and pepper.

Sautéed Carrots,
Asparagus & Peas,
recipe on
page 134 »

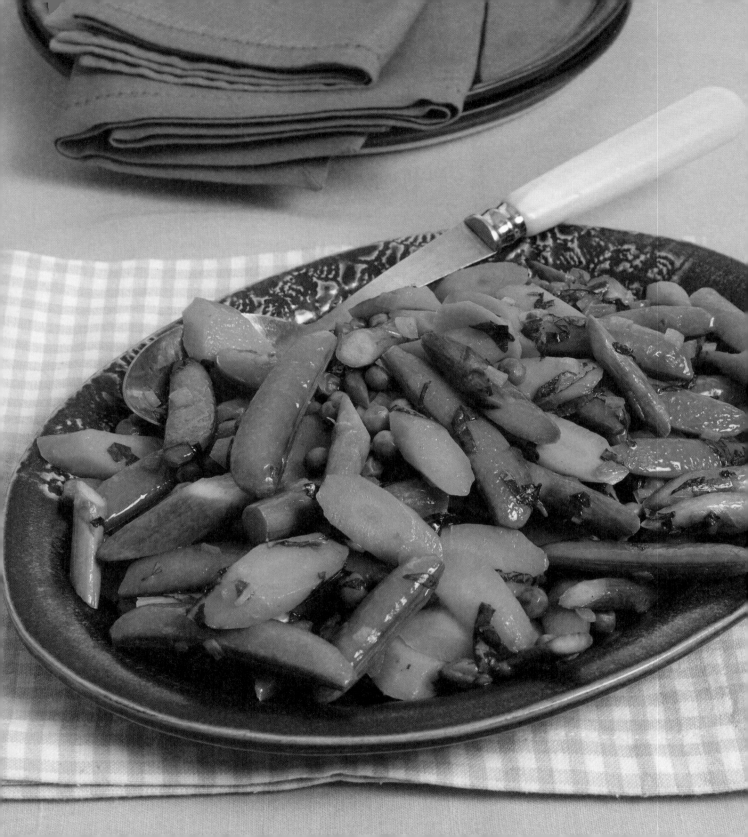

Sautéed carrots and peas are a tried-and-true classic; here the basil and asparagus add a springtime touch and an earthy flavor that amps up the traditional dish. You can also add fiddlehead ferns if they are in season. Simply wash and trim the brown parts before adding them to the pan along with the other vegetables.

Sautéed Carrots, Asparagus & Peas

(pictured on page 133)

Serves 6

3 tablespoons extra-virgin olive oil or salted butter

3 shallots, chopped

1 pound asparagus, trimmed and cut into 1-inch pieces

1 pound carrots, cut into matchsticks

1 pound English peas (thawed if frozen)

1 cup fresh basil, thinly sliced

Sea salt

Freshly ground black pepper

1. Heat the oil in a medium sauté pan over medium-low heat. Add the shallots and sauté until soft, 4 to 5 minutes.

2. Add the asparagus and carrots, and sauté until fully cooked, about 6 minutes. You may need to lower the heat and cover the pan to allow the vegetables to cook fully.

3. Add the thawed peas and cook an additional 3 to 5 minutes.

4. Add the basil, salt, and pepper and mix well.

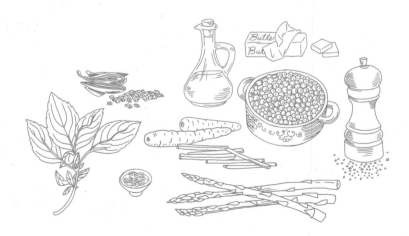

Honeynut squash, which is a smaller, sweeter version of butternut, has become my new favorie squash to cook. I find the taste of honeynut more delicate and subtle than that of larger squashes.

Braised Honeynut Squash with Olive & Prune Relish

Serves 6

FOR THE SQUASH

1 1/2 cups vegetable broth

2 tablespoons salted butter

Sea salt

2 pounds honeynut squash, peeled and cut into 1/2-inch wide strips

Freshly ground black pepper

FOR THE RELISH

1/3 cup coarsely chopped prunes

2/3 cup coarsely chopped pitted green or black olives

1 shallot, finely chopped

2 tablespoons extra-virgin olive oil

1 tablespoon red wine vinegar

1/2 teaspoon anise seeds (optional), slightly crushed in a mortar

Sea salt

Freshly ground black pepper

COOK THE SQUASH

1. Cut a piece of parchment paper into a circle the size of a 12-inch sauté pan, then cut a small hole, about 2 inches in diameter, in the center. Note: this step is optional but it helps to keep the steam in the pan so both sides of the squash cook evenly.

2. Bring the broth, butter, and salt to a simmer in the sauté pan over medium heat. Add the squash and place the parchment round on top. Cover the pan with a lid, reduce the heat to low, and cook for 15 to 20 minutes.

3. Remove the lid and the parchment paper. Increase the heat and boil until almost all the broth has evaporated and the squash is tender but not mushy, 10 to 15 minutes. Season with salt and pepper.

MAKE THE RELISH

1. In a small bowl, combine all the ingredients, mix well, and serve on top of the squash.

My usual way to cook squash is in a soup or roasted with other root vegetables. One day, I decided to try sautéing it and I was happily surprised with the results. The addition of the crisp sage leaves is an obvious one, because squash and sage are a classically delicious combination.

Sautéed Squash with Crisp Sage Leaves

Serves 6

3 tablespoons salted butter

2 shallots, thinly sliced

1 butternut, honeynut, or kuri squash, peeled and cut into 1/2-inch cubes (4 to 6 cups)

3/4 cup vegetable broth

Sea salt

Freshly ground black pepper

4 tablespoons olive oil

10 to 12 fresh sage leaves

1. Melt the butter in a large sauté pan over medium heat. Add the shallots and sauté until soft, about 2 minutes.

2. Add the squash and sauté until lightly browned on all sides, 8 to 10 minutes.

3. Add the vegetable broth. Cover, reduce the heat to low, and cook until the squash is soft and the liquid has mostly evaporated, 5 to 7 minutes. Remove from the heat, season with salt and pepper, and set aside.

4. In a small sauté pan, heat the oil. When hot, fry the sage leaves in batches, for 5 to 10 seconds, until light brown and crisp. Do not crowd them and do not leave them in for too long or they will burn.

5. Remove the sage with a slotted spoon and transfer to a paper towel to drain. When all the leaves are fried, sprinkle them with sea salt.

6. Serve the squash garnished with sage leaves.

Sautéed carrots are my go-to option when I just don't know what else to make as a side dish. Here, I've combined them with kale and broccoli, but they could easily be paired with another sturdy winter vegetable, such as parsnips and chard, or turnips.

Sautéed Kale, Carrots & Broccoli

Serves 6 to 8

Sea salt

1 bunch broccoli, cut into florets

3 tablespoons extra-virgin olive oil

1 large red onion, chopped

6 carrots, peeled and sliced on the diagonal into 1/4-inch slices

2 bunches of kale, stems removed and leaves coarsely chopped

Freshly ground black pepper

1. Bring a large pot of salted water to a rapid boil. Meanwhile, prepare a medium bowl of ice water. Boil the broccoli for 3 to 4 minutes. Drain, and immediately transfer to the ice water for 1 to 2 minutes. Drain and set aside.

2. Heat the oil in a large sauté pan over medium heat. Add the onion and sauté until soft, 2 to 3 minutes.

3. Add the carrots and sauté for 2 minutes. Cover, reduce the heat to low, and cook until just soft, for 5 to 7 minutes.

4. Uncover the pan, add the broccoli and kale, and sauté until the kale is just wilted, 2 to 3 minutes.

5. Remove from the heat and season with salt and pepper.

This dish goes well with the Quinoa "Fried Rice" recipe on page 117, or even with a simple bowl of brown rice. Feel free to experiment with different mushrooms, such as cremini, or a combination of several types.

Stir-Fried Shiitake Mushrooms with Celery & Ginger

Serves 6

1 tablespoon olive oil

1-inch piece of fresh ginger, peeled and cut into matchsticks

4 celery stalks, sliced on the diagonal into 1/4-inch pieces

6 scallions, thinly sliced (white and green parts separated)

8 ounces shiitake mushrooms, stems removed and caps thinly sliced (about 2 cups)

Sea salt

Freshly ground black pepper

1. Heat a large sauté pan over medium heat. Pour in the oil and swirl it around to coat the sides of the pan.

2. Add the ginger and stir-fry until fragrant, about 30 seconds. Add the celery and the white parts of the scallions and stir-fry for 1 minute.

3. Add the mushrooms and cook, stirring frequently, for 2 to 3 minutes.

4. Add 1 tablespoon of water and season the mixture with salt and pepper. Cover, reduce the heat to low, and cook for another 2 minutes, until the vegetables are tender. Garnish with the green parts of the scallions and serve.

A close friend of mine gave me this recipe. She serves this dish every year at Diwali — the Festival of Lights — and I love it! The tamarind gives the squash a nice kick.

Kaddu Bharta with Tamarind

Serves 6 to 8

2 tablespoons ghee or butter

1 dried Indian red chile*

1 teaspoon black mustard seeds

1-inch piece of fresh ginger, peeled and grated

1 teaspoon fennel seeds

1 teaspoon cumin seeds

1 teaspoon fenugreek seeds

1/8 teaspoon cayenne pepper

2 medium butternut squash, peeled and cut into 1-inch cubes

3 tablespoons tamarind pulp*, soaked in hot water to soften

1 teaspoon Sucanat* or brown sugar

Sea salt

Freshly ground black pepper

1/4 cup chopped fresh cilantro

1. Heat the ghee in a large pot over medium heat. Add the chile and mustard seeds. When the seeds start popping, stir in the grated ginger, the fennel, cumin, and fenugreek seeds, and the cayenne. Sauté for 1 minute.

2. Add the squash and 1/4 to 1/2 cup of water. Cover, reduce the heat to low, and simmer until the squash is very soft, 20 to 30 minutes. Remove half of the squash from the pan and place in a large bowl. Mash it with a potato masher. Return it to the pan.

3. Add the tamarind pulp and Sucanat to the pan with the squash. Mix well and cook until heated through, about 5 minutes.

4. Remove from the heat and season with salt and pepper. Garnish with cilantro.

*NOTES: Dried Indian red chile, tamarind pulp, and Sucanat (which is a dehydrated cane sugar), and can be found in most specialty food stores or online.

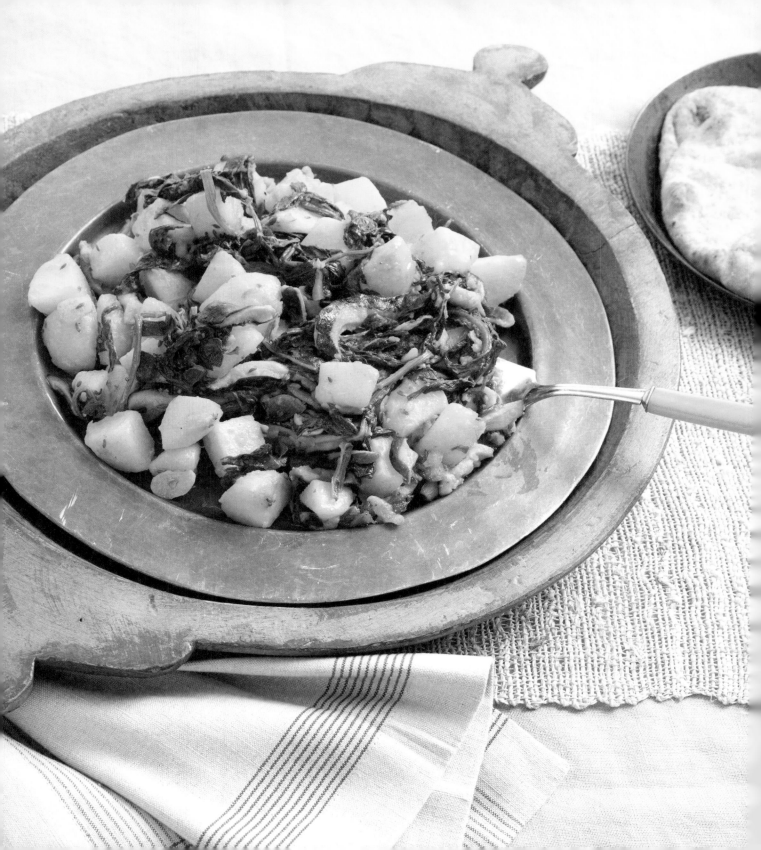

I love the combination of mushrooms and spinach and would happily eat it all year long. I would recommend serving this dish with basmati rice and dal. Alternatively, it can be served on toast for a hearty breakfast or lunch.

Indian-Style Spinach, Mushrooms & Potatoes

Serves 6 to 8

8 tablespoons ghee or butter

8 ounces mushrooms, sliced 1/4 inch thick

Sea salt

Freshly ground black pepper

1 pound spinach, thick stems trimmed

1 teaspoon cumin seeds

4 garlic cloves, thinly sliced

1/2 teaspoon ground turmeric

4 medium waxy (Yukon Gold) potatoes, boiled, peeled, and cut into 1/2-inch cubes

1. Heat 2 tablespoons of the ghee in a large sauté pan over medium heat. Add the mushrooms and cook until browned, about 7 minutes. Season with salt and pepper. Transfer the mushrooms to a medium bowl.

2. Wipe the pan clean and add 2 more tablespoons of the ghee. Heat over medium heat. Add the spinach and a pinch of salt and sauté until the spinach leaves are wilted and the liquid has evaporated, about 5 minutes. Add the spinach to the bowl with the mushrooms.

3. Wipe the pan clean again and add the remaining 4 tablespoons ghee. When melted, add the cumin seeds. When the seeds begin to pop, stir in the garlic and turmeric. Sauté for 30 seconds, then add the potatoes.

4. Sauté the potatoes until lightly browned on all sides, 7 to 10 minutes. Return the spinach and mushroom mixture to the pan and mix well.

I came up with this recipe when I had some leftover mashed potatoes and spinach from the night before and I wanted to liven them up for the family. Served with a freshly made mayonnaise or aïoli, they are absolutely delicious.

Potato, Celery Root & Spinach Patties with Aïoli

Serves 6 to 8

3/4 pound russet potatoes, peeled and cubed

3/4 pound celery root, peeled and cubed

1/2 cup whole, raw milk (pasteurized can be substituted)

2 tablespoons salted butter

Sea salt

Freshly ground black pepper

1/2 cup extra-virgin olive oil, more as needed

1 medium onion, chopped

1 garlic clove, chopped

1/2 pound spinach, thick stems trimmed, leaves coarsely chopped

2 large eggs

1/4 cup all-purpose flour

1 cup grated Parmigiano-Reggiano

Paprika Aïoli (recipe follows)

1. Cover the potatoes and celery root with cold water in a large pot and bring to a boil. Boil 20 to 25 minutes, until soft. Drain. Return the potatoes and the celery root to the pot.

2. Add the milk and butter and mash until smooth. Season with salt and pepper. Transfer the mixture to a medium bowl and let cool.

3. Heat 2 tablespoons of the oil in a large sauté pan over medium heat. Add the onion and garlic and sauté until soft, 3 to 5 minutes.

4. Add the spinach and sauté until wilted, about 3 minutes. Season with salt and pepper. Add the spinach to the potato and celery root mixture and mix well. Wipe the pan clean.

5. Add the eggs, flour, and cheese to the potato mixture and mix well—it should resemble a thick dough. Form the mixture into 2-inch-wide patties and place on a baking sheet. You should have about twelve 1-inch-thick patties.

4. Heat 4 tablespoons of the oil over medium to high heat in the pan used to sauté the spinach. Place several patties in the pan, being careful not to put them too close together, as you will need to flip them. Cook until brown on each side, 3 to 4 minutes per side. Repeat with the remaining oil and the rest of the patties. Serve with paprika aïoli.

Paprika Aïoli

Makes about 2 cups

2 large egg yolks, at room
   temperature

3 garlic cloves garlic, grated

1 1/2 tablespoons white-wine
   vinegar

2 cups extra-virgin olive oil

Sea salt

Freshly ground black pepper

1/4 teaspoon smoked paprika

Pinch of cayenne pepper

1. Combine the egg yolks, garlic, and vinegar in a large bowl.
   Whisk until the mixture is foamy.

2. Slowly pour in the oil, a few drops at a time, whisking continuously in the same direction until the mixture thicens to the consistency of mayonnaise, 3 to 5 minutes.

3. Season with salt, pepper, smoked paprika, and cayenne pepper
   to taste and mix well.

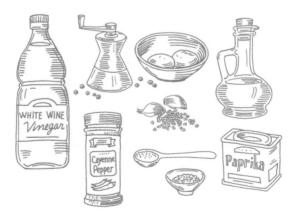

Preserved lemon is typical of Northern African cuisine.
Though less tart, it is more intense and complex than fresh lemon
and works to lift the flavors of the other ingredients in the dish.

Sautéed Onions, Carrots, Fennel & Cabbage with Preserved Lemons

Serves 6 to 8

6 tablespoons salted butter

2/3 cup chopped shallots or
    spring onions

1 leek, white and light-green parts
    only, thinly sliced, then soaked in
    cold water to remove the grit

1 medium red onion, thinly sliced

4 carrots, cut into matchsticks

1 fennel bulb, cut into matchsticks

1 small head of green cabbage
    (about 1 pound), shredded

2 tablespoons chopped preserved
    lemon* plus 1 tablespoon brine

1 teaspoon crushed red pepper
    flakes

Sea salt

Freshly ground black pepper

2 tablespoons chopped fresh parsley

1. Melt the butter in a large sauté pan over medium heat.

2. Add the shallots or spring onions, leeks, and red onion and sauté until soft. Add the carrots, fennel, and cabbage and sauté an additional 2 to 3 minutes. Cover, reduce the heat to low, and cook until the carrots and fennel are soft, 5 to 7 minutes.

3. Stir in the preserved lemon and brine, red pepper flakes, salt, and pepper. Cook another 2 to 3 minutes.

4. Garnish with parsley.

*NOTE: Preserved lemon can be found in most specialty stores or online.

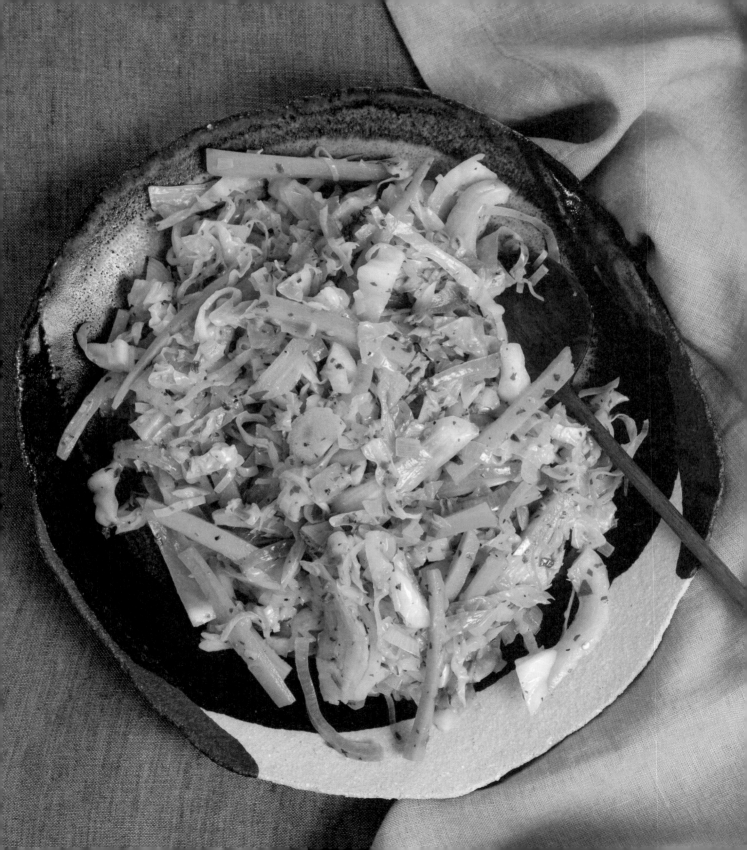

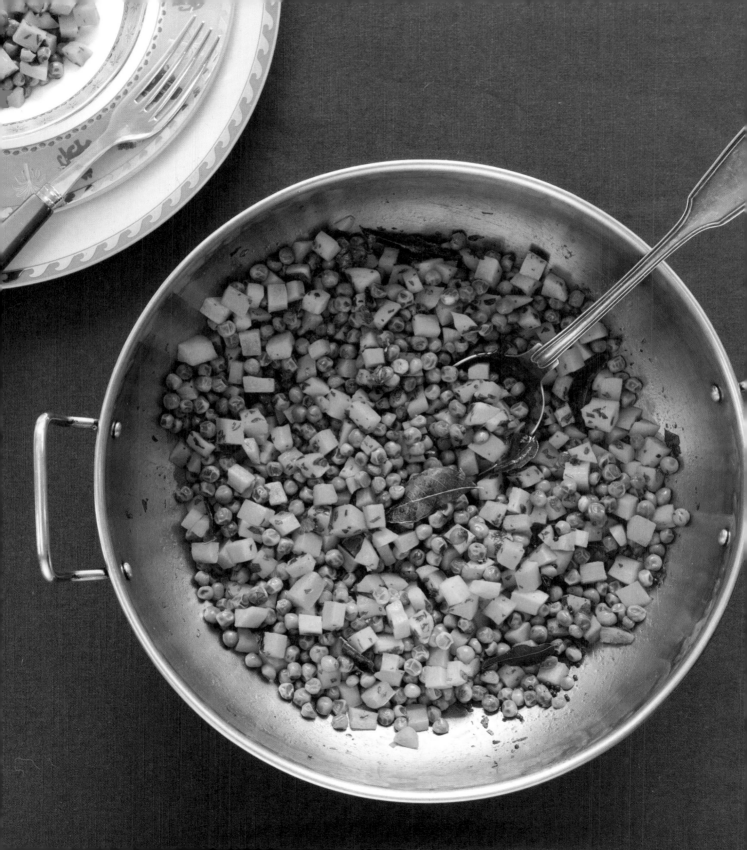

This dish is a variation on traditional peas and carrots. It goes well with plain rice and Indian-Spiced Meatballs (see page 99).

Mattar-Gaajar

Serves 6

2 tablespoons ghee or butter

I teaspoon black mustard seeds

I teaspoon ground turmeric

I teaspoon curry powder

20 curry leaves* (optional)

2 cups frozen peas, thawed

2 cups 1/4-inch-diced carrots

Sea salt

1/4 cup chopped fresh cilantro

1. Melt the ghee in a large sauté pan over medium heat. Add the mustard seeds.

2. When the seeds start popping, reduce the heat and add the turmeric, curry powder, curry leaves, peas, and carrots. Mix well and cook for 5 minutes.

3. Add 1/4 cup of water and salt and bring to a simmer. Cover the pan, reduce the heat to low and cook until the carrots are tender, 8 t0 10 minutes.

4. Uncover, stir in the cilantro, and serve.

*NOTE: Curry leaves can be found in most specialty Indian stores or online.

This is a delicious dish to prepare when you've got a bounty of zucchini and summer squash. While neither of these vegetables is typically used in Indian cuisine, the spices in this dish give it a distinctly Indian flavor, making it the perfect accompaniment to any of the other Indian-inspired dishes in this book.

Cumin-Spiced Summer Vegetables

Serves 6

3 tablespoons ghee or salted butter

2 teaspoons cumin seeds

2 teaspoons black mustard seeds

2 dried Indian red chiles*

2 medium red onions, chopped

3 red bell peppers, seeded and cut into 1/4-inch cubes

2 zucchini, cut into 1/4-inch cubes

2 yellow squash, cut into 1/4-inch cubes

2 ears of corn, kernels cut off the cob

1/4 cup chopped fresh cilantro

Sea salt

Freshly ground black pepper

1. Melt the ghee in a large sauté pan over medium heat. Add the cumin and mustards seeds.

2. When the seeds start popping, reduce the heat to low and add the dried chiles. As soon as the chiles swell and darken, add the onions to the pan. Sauté the onions until soft, about 3 minutes.

3. Add the red pepper, zucchini, and yellow squash and continue to cook until soft, stirring occasionally, 3 to 5 minutes. Add the corn and cook 2 minutes longer.

4. Stir in the cilantro, season with salt and pepper, and serve.

*NOTE: Dried Indian red chiles can be found in most specialty food stores or online.

Combined with a salad or some sautéed greens, this gratin makes for a satisfying vegetarian meal. You can prepare any variation of vegetable gratins in this way. Try combining potato and sunchoke or sweet potato.

Root Vegetable Gratin

Serves 6 to 8

3 tablespoons butter, plus more for the baking dish

3 cups heavy cream

1 teaspoon paprika

1/4 teaspoon ground nutmeg

Dash of Tabasco sauce (optional)

3 leeks, white and light-green parts only, thinly sliced, then soaked in cold water to remove the grit

2 tablespoons fresh thyme leaves

Sea salt

Freshly ground black pepper

1 1/2 pounds butternut squash, cut from the neck only, peeled and sliced 1/8 inch thick*

1 pound celery root, peeled and sliced 1/8 inch thick

1 pound sweet potato, peeled and sliced 1/8 inch thick

1 pound purple and white potatoes, or white potatoes only, peeled and sliced 1/8 inch thick (keep in a bowl of cold water until ready to use)

2 to 3 cups grated Gruyère cheese

1. Heat the oven to 400°F. Butter a 9x13-inch glass baking dish.

2. Put the heavy cream, paprika, nutmeg, and Tabasco, if using, in a small pan and heat to a simmer over medium-low heat. Remove from the heat as soon as it starts to simmer.

3. Melt the butter in a small sauté pan. Add the leeks and sauté over low heat until soft but not browned, 5 to 7 minutes. Add the thyme and season with salt and pepper.

4. Spread one-quarter of each of the squash, celery root, sweet potatoes, and purple and white potatoes in the baking dish in an even layer. Top with one-quarter of the leeks. Pour in one-quarter of the heavy cream, and sprinkle one-quarter of the cheese on top. Repeat until you have four layers of root vegetables, with the final quarter of cheese on top. Cover the dish with foil.

5. Bake for 30 minutes. Remove the foil and continue baking until the top is browned and the vegetables are soft when pierced with a knife, another 15 to 20 minutes.

6. Let cool for 5 to 10 minutes before serving.

*NOTE: Buy enough squash to yield 1 1/2 pounds from the neck.

Desserts

I am not a big fan of baking, but my friends know that my favorite time of the day is around 4 o'clock when I have a cup of tea and a cookie or a slice of tea cake. While I enjoy the occasional chocolate cake or cream-filled pastry, I tend to prefer lighter cakes made with fruit.

My Grandmother's Apple Tart, recipe on page 158 ››

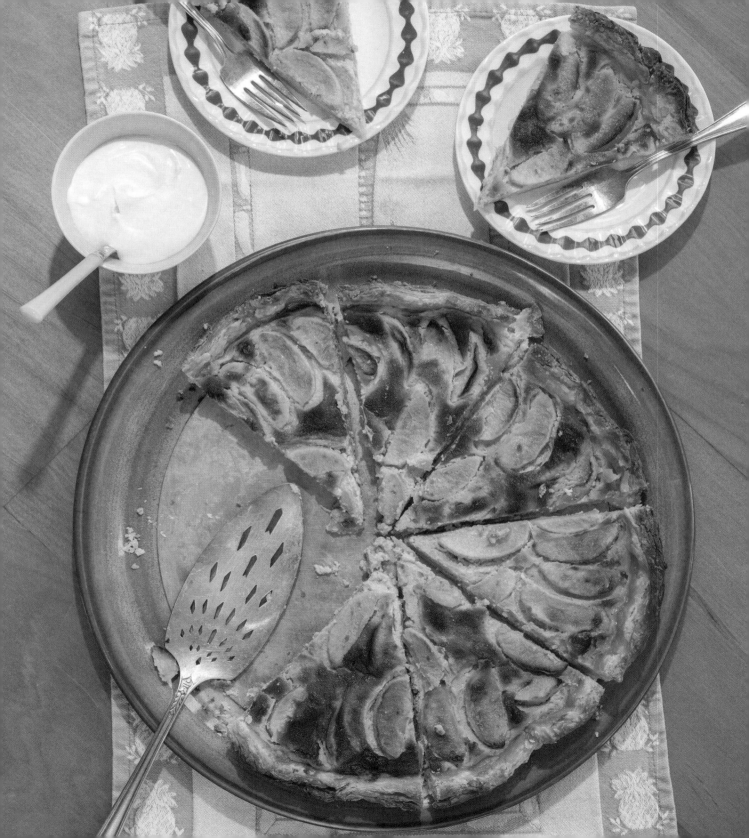

The Formula: **Pound Cake**

I love pound cake anytime of day—for breakfast with some butter and jam, for an afternoon snack with a cup of tea, or for dessert. Mixed berries dress up the cake nicely and the whole-wheat flour gives it a healthier twist. **Makes 1 loaf**

1. Choose the flavor

whole-wheat classic pound cake
chocolate-coffee pound cake
almond and cardamom pound cake
orange-semolina pound cake

2. Gather the ingredients

for the Classic Pound Cake:

2 cups unsalted butter, plus more for the pans
1 1/2 cups Sucanat (dehydrated sugar cane juice)*
4 large eggs
2 cups organic whole-wheat pastry flour
1 teaspoon baking powder
1 teaspoon salt
Zest of 1 lemon
1 1/2 teaspoons pure vanilla extract

for the Chocolate-Coffee Pound Cake:

Replace the whole-wheat pastry flour with
1 1/2 cups all-purpose flour and 1/2 cup
unsweetened cocoa powder
Omit the lemon zest and vanilla extract
Add 1 cup semisweet chocolate chips
Add 1 teaspoon espresso powder

for the Almond-Cardamom Pound Cake:

Replace the whole-wheat pastry flour with
1 1/2 cups all-purpose flour and 1/2 cup almond flour
Replace the Sucanat with granulated sugar
Omit the lemon zest and vanilla extract
Add 1 teaspoon ground cardamom
Add 1 1/2 teaspoons almond extract

for the Orange-Semolina Pound Cake:

Replace the whole-wheat pastry flour with
1 1/2 cups all-purpose flour and 1 cup finely ground
semolina flour
Replace the Sucanat with granulated sugar

Omit the lemon zest and vanilla extract
Add 1 teaspoon orange zest
Add 1 1/2 teaspoons orange blossom water*

3. Make the cake

1. Preheat the oven to 350°F. Butter one 9x5-inch loaf pan.

2. In a stand mixer fitted with the paddle attachment, mix the butter on medium speed until light and creamy. Add the sugar and continue mixing until fluffy.

3. Reduce the speed to low and add the eggs, one at a time, beating until incorporated.

4. In a medium bowl, whisk the flour, baking powder and salt. Add to the butter mixture in 2 additions, mixing just until combined.

5. Remove from the stand mixer and using a rubber spatula, fold in the remaining ingredients.

6. Pour the batter evenly into the baking pan and bake for 45 to 60 minutes, until a toothpick inserted in the center comes out clean. (If the top browns before the cake is cooked through, cover with foil and continue baking until done).

7. Serve the cake with crème fraîche, whipped cream, jam or marmalade, mixed berries, or fruit compote.

*NOTE: Sucanat and orange blossom water are available at most specialty food stores and online.

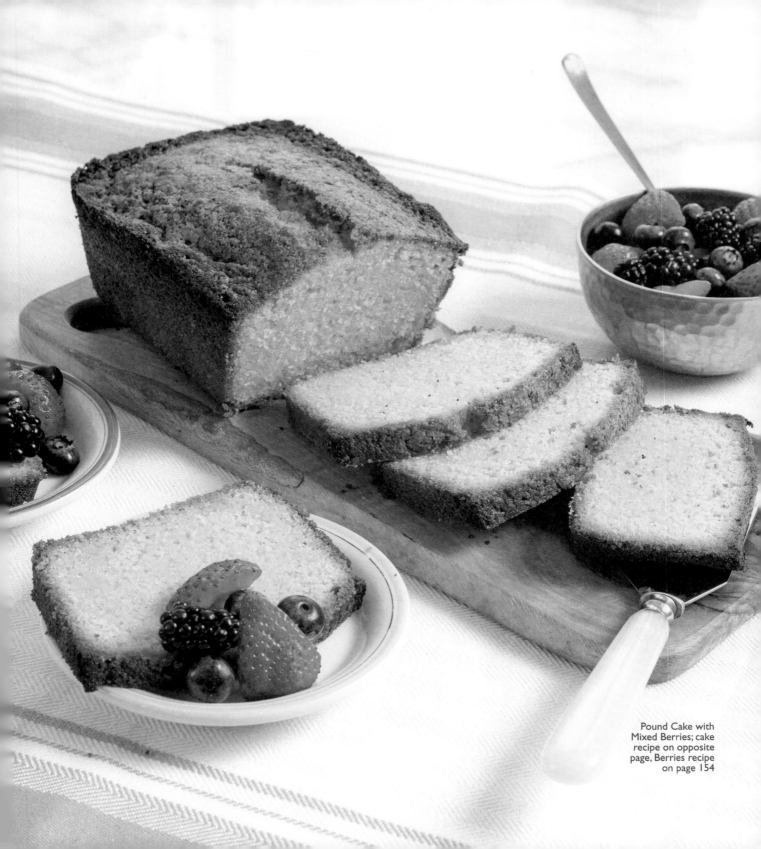

Pound Cake with
Mixed Berries; cake
recipe on opposite
page, Berries recipe
on page 154

Cherry Compote

Makes 1 to 1 1/2 cups

1/2 cup maple sugar

3 tablespoons kuzu root starch *

2 1/2 pounds cherries, pitted,
  juice from pitting cherries reserved

1. Combine the maple sugar, kuzu root starch,
   1 1/2 cups water, and the cherry juice in a small
   saucepan. Whisk over low heat until the kuzu
   starts to dissolve.

2. Add the cherries, increase the heat to medium,
   and bring to a boil.

3. Boil until the cherries are soft and the sauce
   has thickened, 3 to 5 minutes. Let cool before
   serving.

*NOTE: Kuzu root starch is available
at most specialty food stores and online.

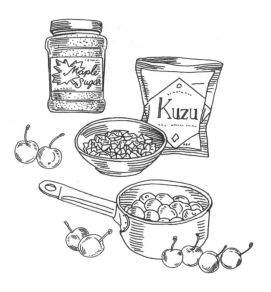

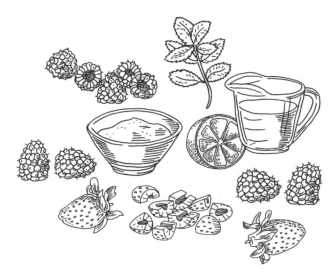

Mixed Berries

Serves 6 to 8

1 quart strawberries, hulled
  and quartered

1 pint blackberries

1 pint raspberries

2 tablespoons granulated sugar

1/4 cup fresh orange juice

2 tablespoons fresh mint leaves,
  thinly sliced

1. In a large bowl, combine all the ingredients,
   mixing gently but thoroughly. Let sit for
   1 hour so the flavors can meld.

Even though I'm not gluten-free, I'm always experimenting with baked goods made with nut flours rather than white flours because nuts are rich in important fats, vitamins, and minerals. Whenever you can substitute Meyer lemons for regular lemons I recommend it. They are a cross between a lemon and a mandarin and, while they have a lemony tang, they are sweeter than regular lemons.

Meyer Lemon Bars with Almond Crust

Serves 8

FOR THE LEMON CURD

Grated zest and juice of 6 Meyer lemons

3/4 cup Sucanat (dehydrated sugar cane juice)*

4 large eggs

6 tablespoons unsalted butter, cut into small pieces

FOR THE CRUST

1 1/4 cups almond flour

1/4 cup Sucanat (dehydrated sugar cane juice)*

1 teaspoon finely grated Meyer lemon zest

1/4 teaspoon sea salt

10 tablespoons chilled, unsalted butter, cut into small pieces

Powdered sugar (optional)

*NOTE: Sucanat is available at most specialty food stores and online.

MAKE THE LEMON CURD

1. In a medium stainless-steel bowl set over simmering water, combine the lemon zest and juice, Sucanat, and eggs and mix well.

2. Add the butter, one piece at a time. Cook, stirring continuously with a wooden spoon, over low heat until the mixture thickens to a curd, 5 to 8 minutes. Strain the curd into a bowl, let it cool to room temperature, then cover with plastic wrap directly on the surface of the curd. Refrigerate for 1 1/2 hours or overnight so the curd can cool and thicken.

MAKE THE CRUST

1. Preheat the oven to 325°F. Line an 8-inch square baking pan with enough parchment paper to leave some overhang on two sides.

2. In a medium bowl, combine the flour, Sucanat, lemon zest, and salt. Mix well.

3. Using your fingers, work the butter into the flour mixture until a crumbly mixture forms. It should come together enough to stick to the bottom of the baking pan. If not, add a little bit of water.

4. Press the dough into the prepared pan. Bake for 30 to 35 minutes to set the crust. Remove from the oven, let cool to room temperature, and then refrigerate for 15 minutes.

5. Pour the Meyer lemon curd over the crust and bake for another 15 minutes, until the curd is set and the crust is lightly browned. Cool to room temperature, then refrigerate until cold. Sprinkle with powdered sugar, if using, and cut the bars into small squares.

I love fruit desserts because they're a great way to use some of the imperfect fruit that might just end up going to waste. While delicious with peaches, you could just as easily make this with nectarines or pears.

Upside-Down Peach & Hazelnut Cake

Serves 8

Unsalted butter for greasing the pan

2 to 3 large, ripe peaches, sliced
1/4 inch thick

2 cups hazelnut flour

5 large eggs, separated

1 cup granulated sugar

1 teaspoon pure vanilla extract

Pinch of sea salt

1. Preheat the oven to 350°F. Butter a 9-inch round cake pan and line the bottom with parchment paper. Butter the parchment paper.

2. Arrange the peach slices in concentric circles around the bottom of the cake pan. Do not overlap the slices.

3. In a medium bowl, using an electric hand mixer, whisk the egg yolks and the sugar until the mixture becomes light and thick. Add the vanilla and mix until well combined.

4. In another medium bowl, using the electric hand mixer (with clean beaters) on medium speed, whisk the egg whites and salt until medium-soft peaks form. Stir half the egg whites into the yolk mixture and mix well. Fold in the remaining egg whites and the walnut flour with a rubber spatula and mix until they are well incorporated.

5. Pour the batter over the peaches in the cake pan. Bake for 40 minutes, or until a toothpick inserted in the center of the cake comes out clean.

6. Let the cake cool in the pan for 10 to 15 minutes, then invert it onto a plate and peel away the parchment paper.

When I was young, my mother made a delicious carrot cake. This recipe is a gluten-
and dairy-free variation on her treasured specialty. It works as well with beets as it
did with carrots. If you like, you can use almond flour instead of hazelnut flour. Be
aware though, that almonds (and, by extension, almond flour) require a lot of water
to produce. Therefore, I recommend using almonds sparingly.

Beet & Hazelnut Cake

Serves 8

Unsalted butter for greasing the pan

4 large eggs, separated

1 cup granulated sugar

2 cups hazelnut flour

1 cup peeled and grated raw beets

1/2 cup dried cranberries or raisins

1 teaspoon lemon zest

1 teaspoon aluminum-free baking powder

Powdered sugar (optional)

1. Preheat the oven to 350°F. Butter a 9-inch springform pan and line the bottom with parchment paper. Butter the parchment.

2. In a large bowl, beat the egg yolks and sugar with an electric hand mixer until light and creamy.

3. In another large bowl, combine the hazelnut flour, beets, cranberries or raisins, lemon zest, and baking powder and mix well. Stir into the egg yolk mixture.

4. In another medium bowl, using an electric hand mixer (with clean beaters) on medium speed, whisk the egg whites to medium-firm peaks and using a rubber spatula, fold them gently into the cake mixture.

5. Pour the batter into the prepared pan and bake for 50 to 60 minutes, until a toothpick inserted in the center of the cake comes out clean. Let cool in pan completely, then unmold onto a serving dish. Sprinkle with powdered sugar, if using.

My aunt recently gave me the recipe for my grandmother's apple tart (which would also be good with pears). It's kind of like a sweet apple quiche and it's delicious served warm!

My Grandmother's Apple Tart

(pictured on page 149)

Serves 8 to 10

FOR THE CRUST

5 1/2 tablespoons unsalted butter, chilled and cut into small pieces, plus more for the pan

1 3/4 cups all-purpose flour, plus more for dusting

1/2 teaspoon sea salt
6 tablespoons ice water

FOR THE FILLING

4 sweet apples (I like to use Fuji or Honeycrisp)

Juice of 1/2 lemon

1 cup heavy cream

2 large eggs

1/2 cup Sucanat (dehydrated sugar cane juice)*

*NOTES:

Sucanat is available at most specialty food stores and online.

You can purchase ceramic baking beans in most specialty cooking stores, or you can just use dried beans.

MAKE THE CRUST

1. Preheat the oven to 400°F. Position a rack in the lower part of the oven. Butter a 10- to 12-inch round tart pan with a removable bottom.

2. In a medium bowl, combine the flour and salt. Work the butter into the flour mixture using your fingers, until a crumbly mixture forms.

3. Add the water and mix until the dough comes together. Flatten the dough into a disk, wrap in plastic wrap, and refrigerate for 30 minutes.

4. On a lightly floured surface, roll the dough out until it is about 1/8 inch thick. Fit the dough into the tart pan (it should go up the sides of the pan). Trim the edges.

5. Prick the bottom of the dough all over with a fork and cover with parchment and baking beans*. Parbake the crust for 15 to 20 minutes.

MAKE THE FILLING

1. Peel, core, and slice the apples into 1/4-inch wedges. Transfer the apples to a medium bowl and mix with the lemon juice.

2. In another medium bowl, combine the cream, eggs, and Sucanat. Mix until the sugar is fully dissolved.

3. Lay the apple slices in concentric circles in the parbaked crust and then pour over the cream mixture.

4. Bake for 30 minutes, until the top is browned and the custard is set. Let cool slightly before serving.

As with the other nut cakes in this section, you can make this cake with any nut flour you like. Walnut flour is another good option. The beaten egg white is what makes the cake so light. You can whip up this gluten-free cake and serve it for dessert, tea, or breakfast. Add some apples sautéed in butter and a dollop of whipped cream for a fancier presentation.

Chocolate-Coconut Hazelnut Cake

Serves 8

Unsalted butter, for greasing the pan

5 large eggs, separated

1 cup granulated sugar

1 teaspoon vanilla extract

4 ounces semisweet chocolate, melted and cooled

2 cups hazelnut flour

1 cup unsweetened shredded coconut

Pinch of sea salt

1. Preheat the oven to 350°F. Butter a 9-inch round cake pan and line the base with parchment. Butter the parchment.

2. Using a stand mixer fitted with the whisk attachment or an electric hand-held mixer, in a large bowl, whisk the egg yolks and sugar until thick and lighter in color, about 2 minutes.

3. Whisk in the vanilla extract. Then add the melted chocolate.

4. In a medium bowl, combine the almond flour and coconut, and mix well.

5. In another large bowl, whisk the egg whites and salt until they hold medium peaks.

6. Stir half of the egg whites into the egg yolk mixture and mix well.

7. Fold the remaining egg whites and half the almond flour-coconut mixture gently into the egg yolk mixture. Fold in the remaining almond flour-coconut mixture. Pour the batter into the cake pan.

8. Bake for 35 to 40 minutes, until a knife inserted in the center comes out clean. Let the cake cool in the pan, and then unmold onto a rack.

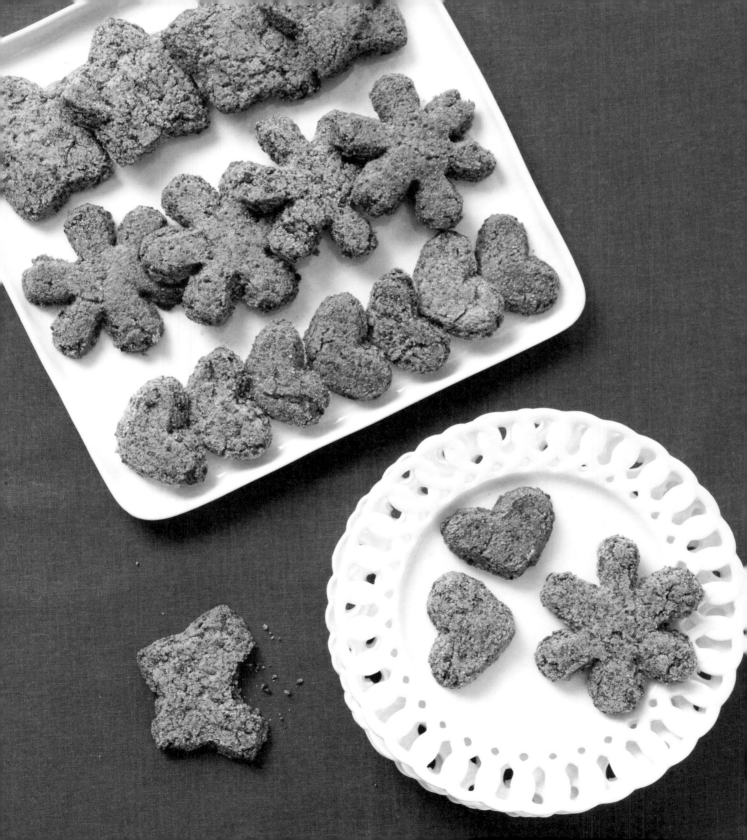

A few years ago, I asked my mother to send me her recipes for holiday cookies so I could start the tradition of baking them with my children. I have fond memories of the scent of chocolate and cloves wafting through the air when my mom made this particular recipe. It's not necessarily a holiday cookie, though the cloves definitely make it more wintry.

Swiss Chocolate Almond Cookies (Basler Brunsli)

Makes 1 dozen cookies

6 ounces bittersweet chocolate, coarsely chopped (about 1 1/2 cups)

1 1/2 cups almond flour*

1 cup granulated sugar, plus more for rolling

1/2 cup powdered sugar, sifted

1 teaspoon ground cinnamon

1/2 teaspoon ground cloves

2 large egg whites

1. In a food processor, pulse the chocolate until it is ground to a crumbly texture (do not overmix or it will melt).

2. In a large bowl, whisk the flour and sugars. Using a wooden spoon, stir in the chocolate. Add the cinnamon, cloves, and egg whites and mix until the dough comes together.

3. Roll the dough into a ball and transfer to a bowl. Chill in the refrigerator for 30 minutes to 1 hour.

4. Preheat the oven to 350°F.

5. Sprinkle granulated sugar on a large wooden cutting board and roll out the dough to 1/2-inch thickness.

6. Line a baking sheet with parchment paper. Using cookie cutters, cut the dough into desired shapes and lay them on the baking sheet about 1 inch apart.

7. Reduce the oven temperature to 325°F and bake for 13 to 15 minutes, until the cookies are slightly firm. Be careful not to overbake the cookies or they will be too hard.

*A NOTE ON ALMONDS: While I like almonds, I am mindful not to use them too much when cooking or baking because they require a lot of water, especially during a drought. In a world where water scarcity is a reality, I try to make food choices that do not worsen the problem.

When I was younger, I remember my mother spending days making traditional Swiss Christmas cookies. Every night it was a different type of cookie. While this recipe was not my favorite when I was younger, it has quickly become popular in my home. Because these need to be left out in a cool, draft-free spot overnight, you need to start preparing them a day ahead.

Anise Cookies

Makes 24 to 30 cookies

5 large eggs

4 cups powdered sugar, sifted

1 tablespoon aniseed, lightly crushed

4 cups all-purpose flour, plus more for rolling

1. In a medium bowl, beat the eggs and sugar until light and creamy.

2. Add the aniseed and flour. Mix well, until the dough comes together fully.

3. Transfer the dough to a wooden cutting board and knead for 3 to 5 minutes, until the dough is silky. Let rest for 10 minutes.

4. Divide the dough into 4 pieces and roll 1 piece on a floured surface to slightly less than 1/2 inch thick. Line a baking sheet with parchment paper. Sprinkle the dough with flour. Using cookie cutters, cut it into desired shapes and lay them on the baking sheet about 1 inch apart. Repeat with the 3 remaining pieces of dough. (If the dough seems dry, put a damp towel over top before the cookies are rolled out.)

5. Leave the cookies uncovered at room temperature in a draft-free area for 12 to 24 hours. The cookies are ready to bake when they feel dry on top and moist on the bottom.

6. When ready to bake, position a rack at the bottom of the oven and preheat the oven to 300°F. Bake the cookies for 12 to 15 minutes, or until the top is firm but the inside is still soft.

I love the combination of chocolate and chestnut, but if you can't find chestnut flour, feel free to use any other nut flour. I like these muffins at teatime but they are equally delicious at breakfast.

Brown Butter Chocolate-Chestnut Muffins

Makes 12 muffins

1 vanilla bean, split lengthwise

1/2 pound (2 sticks/1 cup) unsalted butter, plus more for the pans

3 tablespoons honey

1 1/2 cups chestnut flour

3/4 cup pastry flour

3/4 teaspoon sea salt

5 large egg whites

1 1/4 cups Sucanat (dehydrated sugar cane juice)*

3/4 cup semisweet chocolate chips

1. Preheat the oven to 350°F. Butter a 12-cup muffin pan or line it with parchment baking cups.

2. Using a sharp paring knife, scrape the seeds from the vanilla bean and put the bean and seeds in a small pan. Add the butter and melt over low heat. Once the butter has melted, raise the heat slightly to medium and let it bubble for 5 minutes, stirring continuously, until it darkens slightly. Remove the vanilla bean. Whisk in the honey.

3. In a medium bowl, whisk the chestnut flour, pastry flour, and salt.

4. In a large bowl, whisk the egg whites with an electric hand-held mixer on medium speed. Add the Sucanat and whisk until well combined and the sugar is dissolved.

5. Using a rubber spatula, fold the flour mixture into the egg mixture, and then stir in the vanilla-butter. Mix until smooth and then stir in the chocolate chips.

6. Fill the muffin cups 3/4 full and bake for 25 to 30 minutes, until a toothpick inserted in the center comes out clean. Let cool completely in the pan.

*NOTE: Sucanat is available at most specialty food stores and online.

These quick and easy healthier brownies go well with a dollop of whipped heavy cream. As I mentioned in an earlier recipe, while I prefer to make my desserts gluten-free, I also try to limit the use of almonds. Feel free to substitute hazelnut, walnut, or macadamia nut flour for the almond flour here.

Almond & Olive Oil Brownies

Makes 12 brownies

Unsalted butter, for greasing the pan

1/2 cup fruity olive oil

1 1/2 cups granulated sugar

1/2 teaspoon salt

3/4 cup unsweetened cocoa powder, sifted

1 teaspoon pure vanilla extract

3 large eggs

3/4 cup almond flour*

1 teaspoon aluminum-free baking powder

1/2 cup bittersweet chocolate chips

1/2 cup chopped walnuts or slivered almonds (optional)

1. Preheat the oven to 350°F. Butter an 8-inch square baking pan.

2. In a medium bowl, mix the oil, sugar, and salt. Stir in the cocoa powder and vanilla.

3. Add the eggs and mix well. Stir in the flour, baking powder, chocolate chips, and walnuts, if using. Pour the batter into the baking pan.

4. Bake for 35 to 40 minutes, or until a toothpick inserted in the center of the brownies comes out clean.

5. Let cool before slicing and serving.

*A NOTE ON ALMONDS: While I like almonds, I am mindful not to use them too much when cooking or baking because they require a lot of water, especially during a drought. In a world where water scarcity is a reality, I try to make food choices that do not worsen the problem.

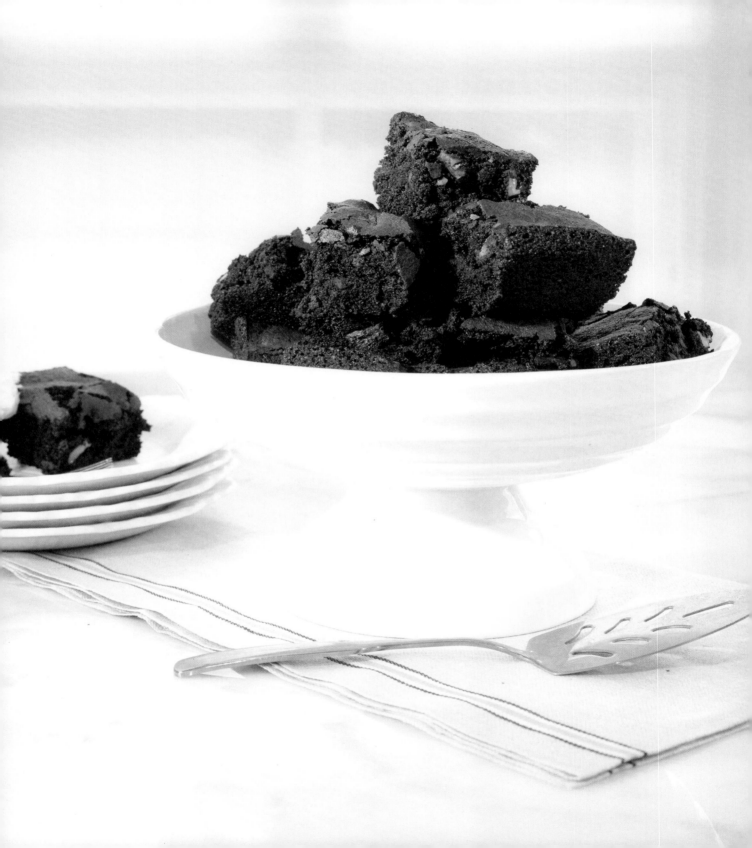

Recipe Index

Resources & Lists

These are my top lists for all things relating to food: movies, books, ingredients, utensils, and more...

My Favorite Dry Goods

Anson Mills
Arrowhead Mills
Bionaturae
Bob's Red Mill grains & flours
Eden Foods
Fig Food Co.
Guittard chocolate
Lotus Foods
Organic Valley
Rustichella d'Abbruzzo

My Favorite Healing Foods

Avocados
Cilantro
Coconut
Eggs
Garlic
Ginger
Lemons
Mushrooms
Onions
Parsley
Pineapple
Sardines

My Favorite Spices & Herbs to Have in the Pantry

Cayenne pepper
Chamomile
Cinnamon
Cumin
Dried dandelion leaves
Echinacea
Nettle
Peppermint
Sea salt
Turmeric

My Favorite Gluten-Free Grains & Flours

Almond flour
Brown rice
Buckwheat
Chickpea flour
Gluten-free oats
Hazelnut flour
Millet
Non-GMO corn
Quinoa

Least Favorite Foods

Any artificially colored candy, especially the red ones
Any highly sweetened cereals, especially the multi-colored ones
Cheetos
Diet Drinks (or anything with artificial sweeteners)
Gatorade
GMO corn and soy
Ketchup
Margarine
Oreos
Wonder Bread

My Favorite Substitutes for White Sugar

Coconut sugar
Date sugar
Honey
Maple syrup
Sucanat (a natural cane sugar made by extracting the juice from sugar cane)

My Favorite Substitutes for Animal Milk

Almond milk
Cashew milk
Hazelnut milk
Oat milk
Rice milk

My Favorite Healthy Fats

Butter & ghee
Coconut oil
Nut oils
Olive oil
Unrefined sesame oil

My Favorite Tools & Equipment to Have in the Kitchen

Cutting board
Electric hand-held mixer
Enamel Dutch oven
Food processor
Good quality chef's knife and paring knife
Measuring cups for wet and dry ingredients
Roasting pan
Stainless-steel mixing bowls
Stainless-steel sauté pan
Wooden spoons, spatula, and ladle

My Favorite Online Resources for Healthy Eating

Directory of CSAs and local food sources
www.localharvest.org

Eat Wild
www.eatwild.com

Environmental Working Group's Shopper's Guide to Pesticides in Produce
www.ewg.org

Heritage Foods
www.heritagefoodsusa.com

Monterey Bay Aquarium Seafood Watch List
www.seafoodwatch.org

Slow Food USA Arc of Taste
www.slowfoodusa.org

My Favorite Food Documentaries

A Place at the Table
Cooked
Fed Up
Food Fight
Food, Inc.
Forks Over Knives
From Paris to Pittsburgh
Look & See
Supersize Me
The Biggest Little Farm
The Future of Food
Wasted! The Story of Food Waste

My Favorite Foodie Movies

Babette's Feast
Big Night
Chef
Chocolat
Eat Drink Man Woman
Jiro Dreams of Sushi
Like Water for Chocolate
Ratatouille
The Hundred-Foot Journey
Tortilla Soup

My Favorite Food Foodie Fiction Books & Memoirs

Gourmet Rhapsody
BY MURIEL BARBERY

Kitchen Confidential
Adventures in the Culinary Underbelly
BY ANTHONY BOURDAIN

Fried Green Tomatoes at the Whistle Stop Café
BY FANNIE FLAGG

Sous Chef
24 Hours on the Line
BY MICHAEL GIBNEY

Delicious!
BY RUTH REICHL

Pomegranate Soup
BY MARSHA MEHRAN

The Last Chinese Chef
BY NICOLE MONES

Lizzy & Jane
BY KATHERINE REAY

Kitchen
BY BANANA YOSHIMOTO

Resources & Lists

Continued from page 169

My Favorite Non-Fiction Food Books

The Third Plate
*Field Notes on the Future
of Food*
BY DAN BARBER

The Unsettling of America
Culture & Agriculture
BY WENDELL BERRY

The Carnivore's Manifesto
BY PATRICK MARTINS WITH
MIKE EDISON

Big Chicken
*The Incredible Story of How
Antibiotics Created Modern
Agriculture and Changed
the Way the World Eats*
BY MARYN MCKENNA

The Hidden Half of Nature
*The Microbial Roots of Life
and Health*
BY DAVID R. MONTGOMERY
& ANNE BIKLE

Salt Sugar Fat
How the Food Giants Hooked Us
BY MICHAEL MOSS

The Gut Balance Revolution
*Boost Your Metabolism, Restore
Your Inner Ecology, and Lose
the Weight for Good!*
BY GERARD E. MULLIN, MD

Soda Politics
*Taking on Big Soda
(And Winning)*
BY MARION NESTLE

Unsavory Truth
*How Food Companies Skew
the Science of What we Eat*
BY MARION NESTLE

Brain Maker
*The Power of Gut Microbes
to Heal and Protect Your Brain —
For Life*
BY DAVID PERLMUTTER, MD,
WITH KRISTIN LOBERG

Grain Brain
*The Surprising Truth About
Wheat, Carbs, and Sugar—
Your Brain's Silent Killers*
BY DAVID PERLMUTTER, MD,
WITH KRISTIN LOBERG

Cooked
*A Natural History of
Transformation*
BY MICHAEL POLLAN

The Omnivore's Dilemma
BY MICHAEL POLLAN

Eating Animals
BY JONATHAN SAFRAN FOER

The Case Against Sugar
BY GARY TAUBES

Bibliography

Barber, Dan. (2014). The Third Plate: Field Notes on the Future of Food. New York: Penguin Books.

Hawken, Paul, ed. (2017). Drawdown: The Most Comprehensive Plan Ever Proposed to Reverse Global Warming. New York: Penguin Books.

Martins, Patrick with Edison, Mike (2014). The Carnivore's Manifesto: Eating Well, Eating Responsibly, and Eating Meat. New York: Little, Brown and Company.

McKenna, Maryn. (2017). Big Chicken: The Incredible Story of How Antibiotics Created Modern Agriculture and Changed the Way the World Eats. Washington, D.C.: National Geographic Partners, LLC.

Nestle, Marion. (2018). Unsavory Truth: How Food Companies Skew the Science of What We Eat. New York: Basic Books.

Safran Foer, Jonathan. (2009). Eating Animals. New York: Back Bay Books/Little, Brown and Company.

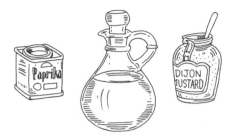

Parting Words

If you are familiar with the October 2018 report by the Intergovernmental Panel on Climate Change, you know that we are well on our way to exceeding the 1.5°C of global warming that the panel warns against and that the increase in temperature will have severe consequences for humanity. I started to consider what I as an individual could do to mitigate climate change, and found myself going back to food because agriculture is responsible for about 11% global carbon emissions (and most likely more if we factor in the effects of deforestation and food waste), and because this was where I felt I could have the most impact.

The goal of this book is to provide a deeper understanding of our food system, and of how our health is delicately intertwined with the health of the planet. If we are to consider regenerating the food system in order to tackle the current climate crisis, we need to stop looking at nutrition, health, and agriculture as three distinct systems. All three systems are highly interconnected and what happens in one affects all the others. This book is meant to serve as a starting point of how we can incorporate the environment in our food choices. As with most things we embark on in life, this is a constant learning process that evolves as our understanding of the ecosystem in which we live deepens. I hope this guide will serve you well wherever you may be on your journey to eating sustainably.

– Rachel Khanna

Notes

Notes

Think Eat Cook Sustainably

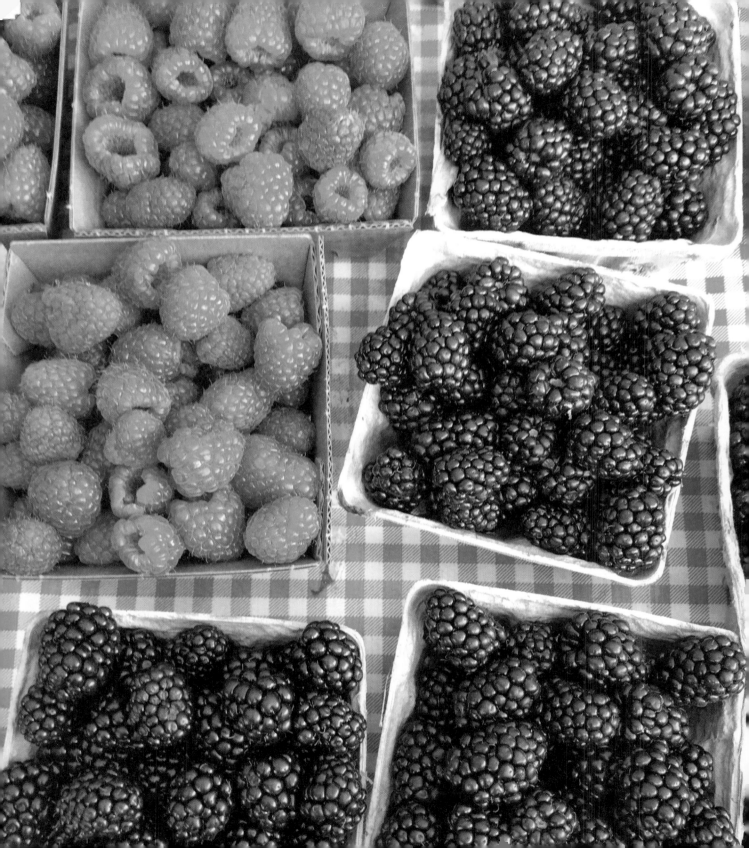